A. Cantrell

D0594231

Motor Speech Disorders

This book is printed on recycled paper. ♻

Motor Speech Disorders

Advances in Assessment and Treatment

edited by

James A. Till, Ph.D.
Speech Laboratory
Veterans Affairs Medical Center
Long Beach, California

Kathryn M. Yorkston, Ph.D.
Department of Rehabilitation Medicine
University of Washington
Seattle, Washington

and

David R. Beukelman, Ph.D.
Department of Special Education and Communication Disorders
University of Nebraska
Lincoln, Nebraska

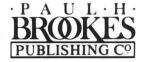
·P·A·U·L·H·
BROOKES
PUBLISHING Cº   Baltimore · London · Toronto · Sydney

Paul H. Brookes Publishing Co.
P.O. Box 10624
Baltimore, Maryland 21285-0624

Copyright © 1994 by Paul H. Brookes Publishing Co., Inc.
All rights reserved.

Typeset by The Composing Room of Michigan, Inc., Grand Rapids, Michigan.
Manufactured in the United States of America by
BookCrafters, Falls Church, Virginia.

Library of Congress Cataloging-in-Publication Data
Motor speech disorders : advances in assessment and treatment/
 edited by James A. Till, Kathryn M. Yorkston, and David R.
 Beukelman.
   p.   cm.
 Includes bibliographical references and index.
 ISBN 1-55766-137-5
 1. Speech disorders. I. Till, James A. II. Yorkston, Kathryn
M., 1948– . III. Beukelman, David R., 1943–
 [DNLM: 1. Dysarthria—diagnosis. 2. Dysarthria—therapy.
3. Voice Disorders—diagnosis. 4. Voice Disorders—therapy. WL
340 M9195   1993]
RC423.M6174   1993
616.85'5—dc20
DNLM/DLC
for Library of Congress   93-13726
                                                                CIP

British Library Cataloguing-in-Publication data are available from
the British Library.

Contents

SECTION I PERSPECTIVES ON MOTOR SPEECH DISORDERS

SECTION II CLINICAL CHARACTERISTICS

Contributors

The Editors

James A. Till, Ph.D., Speech Research Laboratory (126), Department of Veterans Affairs Medical Center, 5901 East Seventh Street, Long Beach, CA 90822

James A. Till is Director of the Speech Research Laboratory of the Department of Veterans Affairs Medical Center, Long Beach, California. He is Associate Clinical Professor and Director of the Speech and Voice Laboratory, Department of Otolaryngology–Head & Neck Surgery, University of California, Irvine. His current work concentrates on computer-assisted evaluation of disordered speech and analyses of diagnostic profiles.

Kathryn M. Yorkston, Ph.D., Department of Rehabilitation Medicine, RJ-30, University of Washington, Seattle, WA 98195

Kathryn M. Yorkston is Head of the Division of Speech Pathology and Professor in the Department of Rehabilitation Medicine and Adjunct Professor of Speech and Hearing Sciences at the University of Washington. Her publications have focused on clinical research in acquired neurologic communication disorders in adults. She has written and edited texts that include *Clinical Management of Dysarthric Speakers*, *Recent Advances in Clinical Dysarthria*, and *Dysarthria and Apraxia of Speech*.

David R. Beukelman, Ph.D., 202F Barkley Memorial Center, University of Nebraska–Lincoln, Lincoln, NE 68583-0732

David R. Beukelman is Barkley Professor of Communication Disorders and Director of the Barkley Augmentative Communication Center, Department of Special Education and Communication Disorders at the University of Nebraska–Lincoln. He is Director of Research and Education of the Communication Disorders Division of the Meyer Rehabilitation Center, University of Nebraska Medical Center. Dr. Beukelman's primary research and clinical interests have been in the areas of dysarthria and augmentative communication.

The Chapter Authors

Scott G. Adams, Ph.D., Speech and Swallowing Laboratory (12-316), The Toronto Hospital, 399 Bathurst Street, Toronto, Ontario M5T 2S8, Canada

Scott G. Adams is a speech scientist/speech pathologist at The Toronto Hospital and the University of Toronto. He received his doctorate from the University of Wisconsin–Madison. His research interests include perceptual, acoustic, and physiologic aspects of the motor speech disorders associated with Parkinson's disease, dystonia, and apraxia. He also maintains an interest in models of normal speech production.

Farhan S. Ahmed, B.S.E.E., M.A., Department of Speech and Language Sciences, Frances Searle Building, Northwestern University, 2299 North Campus Drive, Evanston, IL 60208-3570

Farhan S. Ahmed is a doctoral student at Northwestern University, where he works as a graduate research assistant in the speech perception laboratory. He received his master's degree from the University of Texas at Austin. Currently, he is studying computer speech recognition using parallel distributed processes.

Charles Bombardier, Ph.D., Department of Rehabilitation Medicine, RJ-30, University of Washington, Seattle, WA 98195

Charles Bombardier is Assistant Professor in Rehabilitation Medicine at the University of Washington. He is an attending psychologist for the Rehabilitation Medicine Service at Harborview Medical Center, where he consults on the Neurosurgical Unit and the Outpatient Rehabilitation Medicine Service. Dr. Bombardier received his doctorate in clinical psychology from Washington State University. He also completed a 2-year medical psychology postdoctoral fellowship at Duke University Medical Center.

Michael P. Cannito, Ph.D., Department of Speech Pathology and Audiology, University of South Alabama, Mobile, AL 36688-0002

Michael P. Cannito is Associate Professor of Speech Pathology at the University of South Alabama, where he teaches a course sequence on the neurologic aspects of normal and disordered communication. Dr. Cannito received his doctorate from the University of Texas at Dallas. His research interests include disordered speech motor control, neurolinguistics, and spasmodic dysphonia.

James L. Case, Ph.D., Department of Speech and Hearing Science, Arizona State University, Tempe, AZ 85287-0102

James L. Case is Professor of Speech and Hearing Science and Director of Clinical Services at Arizona State University. He received his doctorate from the University of Utah. His research interests are in voice and the clinical management of voice disorders, cranio-facial disorders, and neuromotor speech disorders.

Carl A. Coelho, Ph.D., Department of Communication Disorders, The Gaylord Hospital, P.O. Box 400, Wallingford, CT 06492

Carl A. Coelho is Director of the Department of Communication Disorders at Gaylord Hospital. His research interests include language and motor speech disorders, and dysphagia secondary to traumatic brain injuries.

Barbara L. Davis, Ph.D., Program in Communication Disorders, Department of Speech Communication, University of Texas at Austin, Austin, TX 78712

Barbara L. Davis is Assistant Professor of Communication Sciences and Disorders at the University of Texas at Austin. Her primary research, clinical, and teaching interests include motor-based characterization of normal speech development and disordered and delayed speech patterns.

Paul A. Dongilli, Jr., Ph.D., Southeast Texas Rehabilitation Hospital, 3340 Plaza 10 Boulevard, Beaumont, TX 77707

Paul A. Dongilli, Jr., is Director of Specialty Programs at Southeast Texas Rehabilitation Hospital in Beaumont, Texas. He received his doctorate from the University of Nebraska–Lincoln. His primary research and clinical interests have involved motor speech disorders in adults with traumatic brain injury.

Drake D. Duane, M.D., Arizona Dystonia Institute, 10250 North Ninety Second Street, Suite 117, Scottsdale, AZ 85258

Drake D. Duane is a neurologist with the Arizona Dystonia Institute and the Institute for Developmental Behavioral Neurology. He is Adjunct Professor in the Department of Speech and Hearing Science at Arizona State University. Before moving to Arizona, Dr. Duane was at the Mayo Clinic, Rochester. His research and clinical interests are in the areas of developmental neurologic disorders, including developmental dyslexia, and dystonia and other movement disorders.

Pinar Ege, Ph.D., Hacetteppe Universitesi, Cocuc Sagugi ve Egitimi Bölumü, 06100 Ankara, Turkey

Pinar Ege is the director of the Speech and Language Clinic in the Department of Child Health and Development of Hacetteppe University, Ankara, Turkey, where she also teaches and conducts research. She received her doctorate from the University of Texas at Austin. Her interests include language development and disorders in children, neurologic aspects of speech and language disorders, and cross-linguistic research.

Marios Fourakis, Ph.D., Department of Speech and Hearing Sciences, 110 Pressey Hall, Ohio State University, Columbus, OH 43210

Marios Fourakis is Associate Professor in the Department of Speech and Hearing Sciences at Ohio State University. His research focuses on the acoustic characteristics of normal and disordered speech.

L. Carol Gracco, Ph.D., Haskins Laboratories, 270 Crown Street, New Haven, CT 06511-6695

A graduate of the University of Wisconsin–Madison, Dr. Gracco is a speech scientist at Haskins Laboratories and Yale University Medical School. Her research interests include the effects of neurologic disease on the vocal tract, with particular emphasis on laryngeal function.

Vincent L. Gracco, Ph.D., Haskins Laboratories, 270 Crown Street, New Haven, CT 06511-6695

Dr. Gracco is Vice President for Research at Haskins Laboratories. He holds a doctoral degree from the University of Wisconsin–Madison. His research interests include sensorimotor mechanisms for speech motor control and articulatory coordination in speech motor disorders.

Mark E. Hakel, M.S., Madonna Rehabilitation Hospital, 5401 South Street, Lincoln, NE 68516

Mark E. Hakel is Director in the Department of Communication Disorders at Madonna Rehabilitation Hospital. He is a doctoral candidate in Communication Disorders at the University of Nebraska–Lincoln. His research and clinical interests are in the area of motor speech and swallowing disorders.

Susan D. Hall, B.Sc., The Heritage School–A Centre for Language and Learning Development, 8540-69 Avenue, Edmonton, Alberta T6E 0R6, Canada

Susan D. Hall is a speech-language pathologist at The Heritage School–A Centre for Language and Learning Development in Edmonton, Alberta. Her work history includes medical, educational, and specialized treatment settings with a variety of special needs populations.

Vicki L. Hammen, Ph.D., Department of Audiology and Speech Sciences, 1353 Heavilon Hall, Purdue University, West Lafayette, IN 47907

Vicki L. Hammen is Assistant Professor of Speech-Language Pathology in the Department of Audiology and Speech Sciences at Purdue University. Her areas of emphasis for research, teaching, and clinical service are motor speech disorders and voice. Dr. Hammen's research interests focus on the relationships between physiologic, acoustic, and perceptual features of both motor speech and voice disorders. She is also interested in the effects of speaking rate reduction on speech intelligibility in Parkinsonian and other dysarthrias.

E. Charles Healey, Ph.D., Barkley Memorial Center, University of Nebraska– Lincoln, Lincoln, NE 68583-0738

E. Charles Healey is Associate Professor of Speech-Language Pathology in the Department of Special Education and Communication Disorders at the University of Nebraska–Lincoln. The author of numerous papers and articles in the field of voice and fluency disorders, Dr. Healey serves as editorial consultant for the *Journal of Speech and Hearing Research* and was the State of Nebraska recipient of the 1985 Clinical Achievement Award for the Advancement of Clinical Practice. He is a Fellow of the American Speech-Language-Hearing Association.

Megan M. Hodge, Ph.D., Department of Speech Pathology and Audiology, 2-70 Corbett Hall, University of Alberta, Edmonton, Alberta T6G 2G4, Canada

Megan M. Hodge is Assistant Professor in the Department of Speech Pathology and Audiology at the University of Alberta and Research Associate in the Department of Communication Disorders at the Glenrose Rehabilitation Hospital in Edmonton, Alberta. Her research interests include developmental aspects of normal and disordered speech production and perception and evaluation of clinical change in children with speech disorders.

Mehdi Jafari, Ph.D., Speech Research Laboratory (126), Veterans Affairs Medical Center 5901 East 7th Street, Long Beach, California 90822

Mehdi Jafari is a research scientist at the Speech Research Laboratory, Veterans Affairs Medical Center in Long Beach/Department of Otolaryngology–Head & Neck Surgery, University of California–Irvine. He has a doctorate in biomedical engineering from University of Texas Southwestern Medical Center at Dallas/ University of Texas at Arlington. His background is in electrical and control systems engineering.

Ray D. Kent, Ph.D., Waisman Center, University of Wisconsin–Madison, 1500 Highland Avenue, Madison, WI 53705-2280

Ray D. Kent is Professor of Communicative Disorders and Coordinator of the Communication Processes Unit at the Waisman Center. He received his doctorate from the University of Iowa. His primary research interests are neurogenic speech disorders, typical and atypical speech development in children, instrumental methods of speech evaluation, and the basic sciences of speech communication.

David P. Kuehn, Ph.D., Department of Speech and Hearing Science, University of Illinois at Urbana–Champaign, Champaign, IL 61820

David P. Kuehn is Professor in the Department of Speech and Hearing Science at the University of Illinois. He received his doctorate from the University of Iowa. His research area is speech anatomy and physiology with a specific focus on the velopharyngeal region.

Leonard L. LaPointe, Ph.D., Department of Speech and Hearing Science, Arizona State University, Tempe, AZ 85287-0102

Leonard L. LaPointe is Professor of Speech and Hearing Science at Arizona State University and Editor-in-Chief of the *Journal of Medical Speech-Language Pathology.* He received his doctoral degree from the University of Colorado–Boulder. His research interests are in cognitive-linguistic interactions, aphasiology, and neuromotor speech disorders.

Cindy B. Law-Till, M.A., 3780 Wisteria Street, Seal Beach, CA 90740

Cindy B. Law-Till is a speech-language pathologist with 10 years of experience treating adults with speech and language disorders. She has coauthored articles appearing in the *Journal of Speech and Hearing Disorders, Journal of Voice,* and *Archives of Otolaryngology.* She currently is a consultant for medical chart review and specializes in third-party payment issues.

Anders Löfqvist, Ph.D., Haskins Laboratories, 270 Crown Street, New Haven, CT 06511-6695

Anders Löfqvist received his doctorate from the University of Lund, Sweden. He is a speech scientist at Haskins Laboratories, working in speech motor control and laryngeal function in speech.

Daryl M. Lorell, M.S., Department of Speech Pathology and Audiology, National Center for Voice and Speech, Laboratory of Speech and Language Neuroscience, University of Iowa, Iowa City, IA 52242

Daryl M. Lorell is a doctoral student in the Department of Speech Pathology and Audiology at the University of Iowa. Her primary research interests are the effects of strength and endurance training on dysarthric speech. Previously, Ms. Lorell worked as a speech-language pathologist at the Cleveland Clinic Foundation, Cleveland, Ohio. She received her master's degree from the University of Wisconsin–Madison.

Erich S. Luschei, Ph.D., Department of Speech Pathology and Audiology, National Center for Voice and Speech, Laboratory of Speech and Language Neuroscience, University of Iowa, Iowa City, IA 52242

Erich S. Luschei is Professor of Speech Pathology and Audiology at the University of Iowa. He is a neurophysiologist who studies the neuromuscular and sensory processes that control the larynx, tongue, and mandible. Dr. Luschei uses experimental approaches in his work, which ranges from the study of tongue strength in normal and disordered speakers to basic neurophysiologic studies of laryngeal control in anesthetized animals.

Kenneth P. Marek, M.D., Department of Neurology, Yale University School of Medicine, 333 Cedar Street, P.O. Box 3333, New Haven, CT 00511

Kenneth P. Marek is Assistant Professor of Neurology and Director of the Movement Disorders Center at the Yale University School of Medicine. His research interests range from the molecular mechanisms underlying neurodegenerative diseases to the clinical and therapeutic aspects of these disorders. Specific studies involve development of mesencephalic neurons in vitro, in vivo imaging in parkinsonian patients, evaluation of nondopaminergic parkinsonian symptoms, and neurotransplantation for parkinsonism.

Thomas P. Marquardt, Ph.D., Program in Communication Sciences and Disorders, Department of Speech Communication, University of Texas at Austin, Austin, TX 78712

Thomas P. Marquardt is Professor of Communication Sciences and Disorders at the University of Texas at Austin. His research interests include aphasia and motor speech disorders in children and adults.

Monica A. McHenry, Ph.D., Galveston Institute of Human Communication, Transitional Learning Community, 1528 Postoffice Street, Galveston, TX 77553

Monica A. McHenry is a speech scientist at the Galveston Institute of Human Communication. Dr. McHenry blends her clinical and research interests through instrumentation-based analysis of the physiologic systems involved in speech production. She is particularly interested in the contribution of physiologic and psychologic variables to intelligibility following traumatic brain injury.

John T. Minton, III, M.S., Galveston Institute of Human Communication, Transitional Learning Community, 1528 Postoffice Street, Galveston, TX 77553

John T. Minton, III, is Computer Research Analyst at the Transitional Learning Community at Galveston. Mr. Minton holds a master's degree in physics from Sam Houston State University. His primary interests are developing software and hardware for data collection and analysis.

Kiyoshi Oshima, M.D., Haskins Laboratories, 270 Crown Street, New Haven, CT 06511 and Research Institute of Logopedics and Phoniatrics, Faculty of Medicine, University of Tokyo, 7-3-1 Hongo, Bunkyo-ku, Tokyo 113

Kiyoshi Oshima is a research staff member of Haskins Laboratories, visiting from the University of Tokyo. He received his medical degree from Tohoku University, Japan. His interests include the electromyographical study of muscles of the vocal tract and their control system during speech.

Donald A. Robin, Ph.D., Department of Speech Pathology and Audiology, Laboratory of Speech and Language Neuroscience, University of Iowa, Iowa City, IA 52242

Donald A. Robin is Associate Professor of Speech Pathology and Audiology at the University of Iowa. He teaches, conducts research, and treats patients in the area of neurogenic communication disorders. His research interests include the measurement of strength and fatigue of oral structures, auditory psychophysics, and attention.

Robert L. Rodnitzky, M.D., Department of Neurology, University of Iowa Hospitals and Clinics, Iowa City, IA 52242

Robert L. Rodnitzky is Professor and Vice Chairman of the Department of Neurology at the University of Iowa College of Medicine and Director of the Movement Disorders Clinic at the University of Iowa Hospitals and Clinics. Dr. Rodnitzky specializes in movement disorders and Parkinson's disease, especially their neuropharmacology and clinical electrophysiology.

Maria Rossetti, M.A., Helen Hayes Hospital, West Haverstraw, NY 10993

Maria Rossetti is a speech-language pathologist in the Head Injury Unit at Helen Hayes Hospital, a rehabilitation hospital in West Haverstraw, New York. Previously, she was a speech-language pathologist at the Rockland County Center for the Physically Handicapped, in New City, New York. She received her master's degree from St. John's University, Jamaica, New York.

Beverly Smith, M.A., Parent Resources for Infant Developmental Enrichment (PRIDE), Department of Mental Health and Mental Retardation, 15800 Highway 620N, Austin, TX 78717

Beverly Smith is a speech-language pathologist for the Parent Resources for Infant Developmental Enrichment program in Austin, Texas. Her clinical and research interests include early communication development in children with developmental delay.

Nancy Pearl Solomon, Ph.D., Department of Speech Pathology and Audiology, National Center for Voice and Speech, Laboratory of Speech and Language Neuroscience, University of Iowa, Iowa City, IA 52242

Nancy Pearl Solomon is Assistant Research Scientist, Adjunct Assistant Professor, and Speech-Language Pathologist at the University of Iowa. She received her doctorate from the University of Arizona. Dr. Solomon's research interests relate to the motor control of speech, especially regarding breathing, phonation, and articulation, in normal and neurologically disordered individuals.

Edythe A. Strand, Ph.D., Department of Speech and Hearing Science, JG-15, University of Washington, 1417 NE 42nd Street, Seattle, WA 98195

Edythe A. Strand is Assistant Professor in the Department of Speech and Hearing Science at the University of Washington. Dr. Strand holds a doctoral degree from the University of Wisconsin–Madison. Her primary research involves the acoustic and physiologic study of motor speech disorders, with a primary emphasis on the dysarthrias associated with neuromuscular disease.

Marsha Sullivan, M.A., Meyer Rehabilitation Institute, Department of Speech-Language Pathology, 600 South 42nd Street, Omaha, NE 68198-5450

Marsha Sullivan is Associate Director of Speech-Language Pathology at Meyer Rehabilitation Institute. Her primary research interests are in motor speech, voice, and head and neck speech disorders.

Jayne M. Wachtel, M.A., Carle Clinic Association, 602 West University Avenue, Urbana, IL 61801

Jayne M. Wachtel is a speech-language pathologist at Carle Clinic in Urbana, Illinois. She is the coordinator of the Cleft Lip and Palate team. Her clinical interests include pediatric voice, speech, language, and feeding disorders. She received her master's degree from the University of Illinois.

Steven Wagner, B.A., Department of Speech Communication, University of Texas at Austin, Austin, TX 78712-1089

Steven Wagner is a graduate student of communication sciences and disorders at the University of Texas at Austin, where he also received his undergraduate degree. He is conducting research on the temporal-acoustic aspects of speech produced with and without concurrent manual signing.

Robin L. Wilson, B.S.N., R.N., Galveston Institute of Human Communication, Transitional Learning Community, 1528 Postoffice Street, Galveston, TX 77553

Robin L. Wilson is a research assistant at the Galveston Institute of Human Communication. Previously, she was a psychiatric research nurse at the University of Texas Medical Branch at Galveston. Her interests include the clinical application of research to enhance patient well-being.

Preface

Motor Speech Disorders: Advances in Assessment and Treatment is written for clinical practitioners in speech-language pathology, researchers in neuromotor speech disorders, and students of neurogenic speech disorders. The breadth of information offered makes the book a valuable resource for other health-related professionals and students as well. The peer-reviewed, original research in this volume represents a broad range of motor speech disorder topics in children and adults. For example, there are chapters reporting speech characteristics and speech-related physiologic functions for individuals with apraxia, spasmodic torticollis, spasmodic dysphonia, traumatic brain injury, and Parkinson's disease.

This book is based on selected papers given at the Conference on Motor Speech Disorders held in 1992 at Boulder, Colorado. The meeting was part of what has now become a decade-long tradition of biennial conferences focusing on dysarthria and other motor speech disorders. The intent of the first Clinical Dysarthria Conference held in 1982 was to draw together clinicians and researchers with interest and accomplishments in the area of dysarthria to present and discuss their most recent work. In order to disseminate that information to a broader audience, selected papers were published the following year in *Clinical Dysarthria*, edited by Bill Berry. Continuation of the conferences at 2-year intervals was fostered by a small core group of people, especially Kathy Yorkston and David Beukelman, who established a loose but very effective organizational structure. These efforts led to other biennial conferences and two other well-received books that disseminated selected papers: *Recent Advances in Clinical Dysarthria* (1989), and *Dysarthria and Apraxia of Speech: Perspectives on Management* (1991).

The previous books and the current volume reflect progressive changes in perspective and advances in knowledge regarding motor speech disorders. Increased accessibility of computers and instrumentation has generated new diagnostic and treatment protocols. Fewer practitioners rely on the ear alone for diagnostic assessment and scientific study. Classification or labeling of persons with motor speech disorders is not seen as the end point of evaluation. Researchers are looking beyond medical diagnosis in order to classify dysarthric individuals for group comparisons. There is increased interest in quantifying functional aspects of the disordered speech related to intelligibility, speech naturalness, and even individuals' attitudes about themselves and their communicative interactions. This book offers readers a valuable update regarding these trends and other information useful for clinical management and research endeavors in motor speech disorders.

Motor Speech Disorders: Advances in Assessment and Treatment is organized into four sections: Perspectives on Motor Speech Disorders, Clinical Characteristics, Advances in Diagnostic Assessment, and Approaches to Treatment. Ray Kent's lead-off chapter in the first section provides an appropriate backdrop for the entire volume. He reviews progress made in describing and understanding motor speech disorders and identifies needs for the future. Chapter 2 by Kathryn Yorkston, Charles Bombardier, and Vicki Hammen provides rare and important information about situational difficulties, perceived reactions of others, and thoughts and feelings of individuals with varying degrees of dysarthria. In Chapter 3, Edythe Strand and Kathryn Yorkston report their results of reviewing subject descriptions in 86 published articles on dysarthria. They make a strong case for considering factors other than medical diagnosis in grouping individuals with dysarthria.

The second section provides valuable descriptive data regarding specific groups of speakers with motor speech disorders. Leonard LaPointe, James Case, and Drake Duane summarize speech and voice characteristics of 70 individuals with spasmodic torticollis. Detailed aerodynamic data for individuals with parkinsonian dysarthria are then reported by Carol Gracco, Vincent Gracco, Anders Löfqvist, and Kenneth Marek. Next is an investigation of acoustic vowel stability in developmental apraxia of speech by Beverly Smith, Thomas Marquardt, Michael Cannito, and Barbara Davis. Michael Cannito, Pinar Ege, Farhan Ahmed, and Steven Wagner report results from diadochokinetic tasks that separate statistically groups of speakers with adductor spasmodic dysphonia, abductor spasmodic dysphonia, and normal speech.

The initial study in the third section illustrates the value of complementary instrumental analyses in diagnostic assessment. Carl Coelho, Vincent Gracco, Marios Fourakis, Maria Rossetti, and Kyoshi Oshima collaborated to report clinically relevant measures of lip-jaw kinematics, vocal tract aerodynamics, and acoustics in an individual with closed-head injury. In the next chapter, James Till, Mehdi Jafari, and Cindy Law-Till report a new accelerometric measure that correlates with listener judgments and differentiates normal and hypernasal speakers. Then, Monica McHenry, John Minton, and Robin Wilson show how articulatory force-testing protocols can be improved for adults with traumatic brain injury. Tongue function testing in Parkinson's disease is the focus of the chapter by Nancy Solomon, Donald Robin, Daryl Lorell, Robert Rodnitzky, and Erich Luschei. They report intriguing differences in strength, endurance, and perception of effort for three subjects with mild parkinsonism. Vicki Hammen and Kathryn Yorkston provide direction for clinical implementation of aerodynamic assessment by documenting the effects of instruction on mean peak pressure and variability. They note important individual differences among their subjects. Paul Dongilli, Jr., then shows that semantic context can have a significant effect on the intelligibility of dysarthric speakers. Comparison of dedicated instrumental and computer systems used to extract fundamental frequency is the focus of the next chapter by Mark Hakel, E. Charles Healey, and Marsha Sullivan. Their findings show acceptable agreement among the systems tested, except for severely impaired voices.

The fourth section of *Motor Speech Disorders* contains three chapters reporting results for specific treatment procedures. First, David Kuehn and Jayne Wachtel report on a highly creative use of continuous positive airway pressure (CPAP) instrumentation to provide resistive air pressure to the velum during exercises designed to improve velopharyngeal closure. The next chapter by Scott Adams provides detailed acoustic and kinematic data describing the effectiveness of delayed auditory feedback for an individual with hypokinetic dysarthria and accelerating speech rate. The third chapter on treatment is by Megan Hodge and Susan Hall. They report a detailed multiphase treatment program developed to increase the speaking rate of an 11-year-old child who suffered a near-drowning accident at age 5.

This book emerged from the effort and cooperation of many individuals. Kathryn Yorkston and co-conference chair Christy Ludlow were very effective in soliciting high-quality submissions for presentation at the 1992 Conferences on Motor Speech Disorders and Motor Speech Control. The program committee for the motor speech disorders papers consisted of Mehdi Jafari, David Beukelman, Kathryn Yorkston, and James Till, chair. The local arrangements for the conference were flawless, thanks to Lorraine Ramig and her team. Once preparation of the manuscript began, the authors of chapters were professional and timely in their production and revision of manuscripts. The many talented professionals at Paul H. Brookes Publishing Co. helped ensure smooth and relentless progress toward publication. Mehdi Jafari was particularly helpful to me at many stages with tracking of deadlines and organization of materials. It is gratifying to know that more people than just those who attended the Boulder conference will benefit from the exchange of information and ideas that occurred.

REFERENCES

Berry, W. (1983). *Clinical dysarthria.* Boston: College-Hill Press.

Moore, C.A., Yorkston, K.H., & Beukelman, D.R. (Eds.). (1991). *Dysarthria and apraxia of speech: Perspectives on management.* Baltimore: Paul H. Brookes Publishing Co.

Yorkston, K., & Beukelman, D. (1989). *Recent advances in clinical dysarthria.* Boston: College-Hill Press.

Motor Speech Disorders

SECTION I

PERSPECTIVES ON MOTOR SPEECH DISORDERS

Chapter 1

The Clinical Science of Motor Speech Disorders
A Personal Assessment

Ray D. Kent

THIS CHAPTER IS an editorial that expresses the author's personal opinion concerning progress in the study of dysarthria and posits a set of recommendations for a research agenda. The opinions pertain to progress in the following areas: clinical taxonomy and nosology, understanding of pathophysiology, assessment and measurement of speech function, understanding of speaker variables as they pertain to motor speech disorders, and clinical management.

PROGRESS IN TAXONOMY AND NOSOLOGY

Progress in taxonomy and nosology has been sluggish—two reasons suggest why this might be so. First, it is possible that taxonomy and nosology are basically complete. Therefore, the systems available account satisfactorily for clinical and research needs, thus obviating motivation for further work. The second possibility is that the area simply has been neglected, although further work on taxonomy and nosology is warranted. The latter seems the more likely conclusion. To a large degree, the Mayo Clinic rating and classification system (Darley, Aronson, & Brown, 1969a, 1969b, 1975a) is the clinical standard, especially in the United States. This system certainly has much to recommend it, but it is not a complete description of the full range of motor speech disorders in children and adults (nor did its originators intend that it be). Some dysarthrias cannot be classified with this system.

Since the Mayo Clinic system was described in published form in 1969, it has not been revised or even supplemented substantially. This system, usually taught in colleges and universities, is the one most often used clinically, and is the one that usually suffices for description of subjects in research studies. (For a recent survey of clinical practice, see Gerratt, Till, Rosenbek, Wertz, & Boysen, 1991.)

The Mayo Clinic system is very good in many respects, and it has fostered a great deal of systematic thinking about the dysarthrias. Indeed, its impact on research and clinical practice has been so profound that if it has *any* weaknesses, efforts should be taken to remedy them. Hence, the question: Is the Mayo Clinic system sufficient and flawless to the extent that at least a modest revision need not be offered? The Mayo Clinic system has survived for more than two decades and perhaps its longevity is evidence enough for its continued value. But a review of the literature reveals some reasons for concern.

One of these concerns is reliability. There have been very few systematic evaluations of the reliability of the Mayo Clinic system. However, one such evaluation (Zyski & Weisiger, 1987) used recorded samples of dysarthria from materials prepared by Darley, Aronson, and Brown (1975b) to determine the accuracy with which classification of dysarthria type was identified by three groups of listeners with varied experience. Listener Group 1 is of particular relevance. These were 17 speech-language pathologists each of whom had a minimum of 5 years of clinical experience and who routinely diagnosed and treated persons with dysarthria. The 17 listeners identified type of dysarthria for 28 recorded samples. Their accuracy was 19%, ranging from a low of 1% for flaccid dysarthria to 55% for hypokinetic dysarthria. Graduate students who received 5 hours of classroom training on perceptual evaluation of dysarthria did better than the professionals. They had an accuracy of 56%, or a little better than half of the samples correctly identified. Perhaps their superior performance reflected the fact that they were trained with the audio seminar materials prepared by Darley et al. (1975b). Zyski and Weisiger (1987) concluded that the Mayo Clinic system was not sufficiently reliable for clinical purposes. This serious negative judgment cannot be ignored. Perhaps in the original studies reported by Darley, Aronson, and Brown, the rating system was sufficiently reliable. What is at question is whether or not the system can be used with adequate reliability by a larger sample of clinicians.

Whatever the status of the Mayo Clinic system itself, the description and analysis of neurologic speech disorders continues to rely heavily upon perceptual techniques such as rating scales. Although rating-scale approaches have been useful for many purposes of description and classification, they have shortcomings. In particular, these methods may suffer from poor reliability for at least some rated dimensions (Sheard, Adams, & Davis, 1991; Zyski & Weisiger, 1987), possible interactions among rated variables (Southwood, 1990), uncertain definition of rated dimensions (Sheard et al., 1991), psychometric unsuitability of some frequently used rating scales for important dimensions of speech—such as intelligibility (Schiavetti, 1992), and limited analytic potential, particularly with respect to phonetic, acoustic, and physiologic correlates of the speech disorder (Collins, 1984; Kent, 1992). Motor speech disorders frequently are described as a collective of perceptual dimensions, and this approach underlies the prevailing systems for clinical categorization and rating of severity. Indeed, perceptual judgment is essential to many purposes, such as evaluating the intelligibility and quality of speech. At present there is no instrumental assessment to scale speech intelligibility (although progress has been made in the application of computer recognition to limited samples of dysarthric speech; Coleman & Meyers, 1991). Moreover, despite many attempts to define instrumental correlates of voice quality disorders, there is relatively little consensus about the selection of measures correlated with perceptual ratings of quality. Difficulties have been summarized by Eskenazi, Childers, and Hicks (1990), Hicks (1992), Kent (1992), Kreiman, Gerratt, and Precoda (1990), Kreiman, Gerratt, Precoda, and Berke (1992), and Wolf and Steinfatt (1987).

What are the prospects for improved evaluations of speech intelligibility and speech-voice quality? Considerable progress has been made in the assessment of speech intelligibility, so much so that dysarthria, speech of deaf persons, and phonological disorders in children may be leading the field of speech pathology in attempts to quantify and explain intelligibility deficits.

Voice and speech quality are particularly important in most perceptual evaluations of dysarthria, and published evidence supports the conclusion that speakers with dysarthria often have impairments of quality (Darley et al., 1975a; Griffiths & Bough, 1989; Kent, 1992). Speakers with dysarthria are often said to have voice quality disorders such as harshness, hoarseness, breathiness, monotonicity, strain-strangled, or inappropriate pitch level. However, determining acoustic correlates of the perceived voice quality impairments in dysarthria has had limited success. Particularly with respect to the perturbation measures of jitter, shimmer, and speech-to-noise (S/N) ratio, some studies of persons with dysarthria-related voice problems do not indicate that these measures have much clinical value (Zwirner, Murry, & Woodson, 1991). Our own results in progress similarly question the value of acoustic perturbation measures in discriminating among clinical subgroups or even in separating clinical groups from control groups. Interestingly, our data suggest that the clinical value of these measures may be greater for women than for men. It seems timely to reevaluate the application of acoustic measures to voice problems in persons with dysarthria. It is questionable if any one acoustic measure, such as jitter, will hold much clinical significance across different types of dysarthrias. An alternative approach is factor analysis, with the aim of determining if a particular combination of weighted acoustic measures will account for perceptual ratings of voice quality in dysarthria. The successful application of factor analysis will depend upon the collection of data for a suitably large number of subjects in different dysarthric subgroups.

The weak association between acoustic measures and perceptual ratings of voice quality reported for subjects with dysarthria has a parallel in other speech and voice disorders, including the speech of persons who are deaf (Arends, Povel, Van Os, & Speth, 1990) and voice disorders (Eskenazi et al., 1990). Wolf and Steinfatt (1987) reported that different acoustic variables were the best predictors for different voice types. Kreiman et al. (1992) observed that expert judges differed considerably with respect to the acoustic factors correlated with their perceptual ratings of pathological voices. These results indicate that a fixed set of acoustic measures will not necessarily correlate highly with perceived severity across a range of vocal abnormalities and across different judges—even experienced judges. This situation would compromise the traditional clinical evaluations of dysarthria severely, because these involve a small number of judges (often one) evaluating several different types of dysarthria (and presumably different voice qualities). It is proper to ask: Can we reasonably expect a set of judges to make reliable and valid perceptual assessments of different voice qualities?

What may be required for the future development of sensitive and effective clinical evaluation is an integration of human perceptual judgment with instrumental evaluation. Orlikoff (in press) stated that a comprehensive assessment of speech function depends upon a balance of physical and perceptual analyses. Exclusive reliance on either one alone may limit the understanding of speech impairments. To a degree, different methods of evaluation are complementary. For example, clinicians' judgments of severity may depend primarily upon the slowly varying components of the temporal pattern of speech and rather less upon rapidly varying temporal features such as stop bursts and voice onset times (Seikel, Wilcox, & Davis, 1990). If such a result has general application, then acoustic analysis of slowly varying temporal properties, such as vowel and consonant durations, could be used to define physical correlates of perceived severity. Acoustic analysis of rapidly varying properties could provide information on the dysarthria that is not readily appreciated by the ear.

However, beyond the effective combination of data from different methods lies the larger question of clinical classification. Rosenbek and McNeil (1991) wrote a challenging paper on the problems of classifying dysarthria and apraxia of speech. Their comments warrant careful study in any reconsideration of clinical taxonomy and nosology.

PROGRESS IN UNDERSTANDING THE PATHOPHYSIOLOGY OF SPEECH MOTOR DISORDERS

Progress in understanding the pathophysiology of speech motor disorders has been modest at best. Early promises of electromyography, movement transduction, and other tools to examine pathophysiology have yielded only a low constant rate of scientific return. There have been few break-throughs, certainly too few to attract wide-scale interest among clinicians. Moreover, it seems that few clinicians make routine (perhaps not even occasional) use of instrumental evaluations (although data on this issue are not readily available, Gerratt et al., 1991, report on the clinical practices of one group of clinicians).

Fortunately, investigators persevere in their search for pathophysiologic correlates of motor speech disorders. However, much remains to be done. The extant data are so limited that it is not always clear what kinds of results are pathognomic rather than artifacts or ephiphenomena. For example, Adams (1990) reported in an x-ray microbeam study that multiple velocity peaks often accompanied articulatory movements in slow-rate productions by nondisabled speakers. As Adams noted, multiple velocity peaks also have been observed in some speech disorders, notably apraxia of speech and Parkinson's disease. Given that many speakers with apraxia of speech and dysarthria speak at a slow rate, the clinical interpretation of multiple velocity peaks is not straightforward. This is not to say their appearance is unimportant, but rather that pathophysiologic interpretation is uncertain. Ziegler (1991) described several such examples and concluded that there are serious limitations in current understanding of the pathophysiology underlying speech disorders. In many areas of study, the available data are simply too limited. There are, however, examples of progress in this area, particularly Putnam (1988).

One particular pathophysiology recently examined by investigators in both speech and nonspeech movement systems is spasticity, and the results of this work are instructive: In the common neurologic description (Lance, 1980), spasticity is related to increased limb tone (clasp-knife type of resistance to passive movement), exaggerated tendon jerks and clonus, Babinski responses in the lower extremities, and impairment of voluntary control of skeletal muscles. With respect to its kinematic properties, spasticity can also be described as a velocity-dependent increase in the tonic stretch reflex. The pathophysiology of spasticity is said to result from a twofold imbalance between excess excitation (e.g., increased phasic stretch reflexes) and deficient inhibition (e.g., suppression of the tonic vibration reflex, reflex irradiation, and abnormal silent intervals in an electromyogram).

Myklebust, Gottlieb, Penn, and Agarwal (1982) reported another neurologic feature in patients with spasticity resulting from perinatal suprasegmental insult. Electromyographic recordings showed that these patients had *reciprocal excitation*, a phenomenon in which segmental stretch reflexes are simultaneously expressed in the agonist, stretched muscle and the antagonist, shortened muscle. This pattern contrasts with the normal pattern of *reciprocal inhibition*, in which the agonist and antagonist have alternating activation of the stretch reflexes. Myklebust et al. concluded that their results require a redefinition of spasticity to include damage to the "immature suprasegmental structure that imposes a secondary, developmental disorder on the spinal cord" (p. 373).

Barlow and Abbs (1984) studied the regulation of fine forces in the oral musculature by subjects with congenital spasticity. The three muscle systems they studied—lips, tongue, and jaw—differ in density of muscle spindles and presence or absence of monosynaptic reflexes. The lips seem to lack spindles, the tongue muscles have a modest number of spindles in some fibers, and the jaw muscles have a comparatively large spindles population. Barlow and Abbs reasoned that if the hyperactivity of muscle-spindle monosynaptic reflexes were a primary determinant of the motor impairment in spasticity, then it would be predicted that the three muscle systems would be impaired to different degrees. The results indicated that, generally, force control was poorest for the tongue and nearly equivalent for the lips and jaw. This result argues against the explanation of impaired orofacial movements in terms of hyperactivity of muscle-spindle monosynaptic reflexes.

Neilson and O'Dwyer (1981) also concluded that hypertonus is not causally related to the impaired speech movements of subjects with cerebral palsy. They suggested that the impairment may be explained better in terms of developmental motor learning (much as Kent and Netsell, 1978, discussed motor learning phenomena related to athetoid cerebral palsy). Neilson and O'Dwyer wrote that if "motor commands are generated on the basis of previously learned correlations between motor events and their sensory consequences. . . , then impairment of sensory-motor integration processes involved in establishing such correlations should disrupt the ability to formulate appropriate motor commands" (p. 1018). The results of Myklebust et al. (1982) also point to a developmental disorder that may contribute to the motor impairment in spastic cerebral palsy.

This brief summary of investigations into the pathophysiology of spasticity points out some basic lessons. First, it should not be asserted uncritically that speech impairments resulting from neurologic disorders can be understood immediately in terms of presumed pathophysiology. Second, the age at onset of the condition may have important implications for understanding the disorder and its effects upon skilled motor behavior. This second point is discussed later in this chapter.

PROGRESS IN ASSESSMENT AND MEASUREMENT OF SPEECH FUNCTION IN SPEECH MOTOR DISORDERS

Progress in assessment and measurement of speech function in speech motor disorders has been substantial, as shown in the following examples.

1. Acoustic analyses that relate abnormalities to underlying system dysfunctions (Hillenbrand & Flege, 1992)
2. Aerodynamic studies that identify locus of disorder and quantify the severity of that disorder (Muller & Brown, 1980; Till & Alp, 1991; Warren, 1992)
3. Perceptual evaluations that inform us honestly of some of the weaknesses as well as the strengths of this approach (Kreiman, Gerratt, & Precoda, 1990; Kreiman et al., 1992; Sheard et al., 1991)
4. Assessments of intelligibility and quality that offer increasingly valid and reliable indices (Kent, 1992; Kent, Weismer, Kent, & Rosenbek, 1989; Weismer & Martin, 1992; Yorkston & Buekelman, 1981; Ziegler, Hartmann, & von Cramon, 1988)
5. Innovative use of techniques to assess strength, fatigue, tremor, rigidity, and reflex status in the oral musculature (Barlow, 1992)
6. Beginnings of the use of brain imaging to establish lesion sites associated with speech motor disorders. (A continuing challenge in the study of speech motor disorders is to explain observed speech impairments in terms of evolving concepts of the neural control of language expression. Careful study of dysarthria and apraxia of speech should expand understanding of the neural regulation of complex behavior. Moreover, study of the speech motor disorders will also be enhanced from a reading of the rapidly growing literature in neural science.)

Effective introduction of these developments in clinical practice depends upon assessment objectives and philosophy. Although the words *measurement* and *assessment* are commonly used, there is no ensurance of uniformity of meaning. Therefore, it may be helpful to define the terms *measurement* and *assessment* as they relate to clinical research and practice, and then to consider one philosophy of assessment. The definitions provided by Kondraske (1989) are particularly apt. *Measurement* is *quantita-*

tion of an observation by the use of a standard, much as the use of a rule to measure length or a thermometer to measure temperature. *Assessment*, as a process, determines the *meaning* of a measurement or a collective set of measurements within a specific context. Assessment also can be viewed as the result of that process.

The distinction between measurement and assessment is important. One can measure, for example, the peak intraoral air pressure associated with a given speech sound. But the task of interpreting the peak value is that of assessment. A reduced oral pressure may reflect several different physiologic events, including impaired pulmonic function, inadequate velopharyngeal valving, poor oral articulation, or a combination of these (Muller & Brown, 1980). In fact, the final assessment may not be based on intraoral air pressure alone but also on other measurements, such as air flow, or on a collective set of aerodynamic measurements.

Netsell (1986) has used the 10-point person effectively as a logical framework for assessment. The assessment goal is to evaluate the functional resources of the various components of the speech production system. The 10 points are not necessarily measurement loci per se. The function of any one point can be determined sometimes by a measurement made at a different location, such as when respiratory function is evaluated by measuring peak inspiratory or expiratory flow at the mouth or nose, or when velopharyngeal function is evaluated by measuring intraoral air pressure behind an oral obstruction. At times we might attempt to monitor the movement of a structure by measuring the effect of that movement on airflow. There is nothing wrong with this procedure as long as it is accomplished with a logical model that relates measurement with its underlying causal event(s). The points are really logic points for assessment and in their collective function they reflect the performance space of speech.

This framework parallels Kondraske's (1989) approach to the general assessment of human performance. Kondraske views the human "as a defined architectural structure composed of a finite set of interconnected functional units capable of operating along specific dimensions of performance." Examples of performance dimensions include strength, endurance, range of motion, and speed. Each functional unit can be mapped onto its own performance space. But when all the functional units are considered, the result is a finite set of distinct basic elements of performance (BEP). The word *finite* is significant because it indicates a limit to the necessary observations. The 10-point person is a finite-set description of BEPs for speech. Thus, it is possible to paraphrase Kondraske as follows for speech assessment: The speech production system is a defined architectural structure composed of a finite set of interconnected functional units capable of operating along specific dimensions of performance. A simple illustration of this structure is given in Figure 1, which identifies the major functional units and indicates the primary interactions among these units by interconnections.

The logic of quantitative clinical evaluation now becomes apparent. Performance is inferred from an assessment logic that determines the meaning of one or more measurements. Quantitation is basic to measurement, but assessment is more than quantitation. It is a logical system that relates observation and allowable inference. It can be the means by which

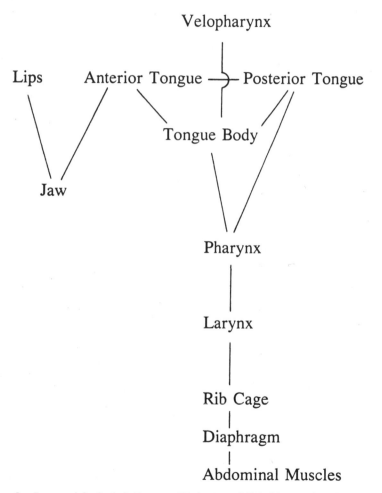

Figure 1. Framework for the Basic Elements of Performance (BEPs) of the speech production system. Each element can be described in terms of kinematic variables such as range, direction, and rate of movement. However, the elements are interactive, because of biomechanical linkages, motor coordination, and participation in a general objective. The lines joining elements indicate some of the interactions of particular importance.

various tasks and measures are integrated in an overall assessment of performance. For example, such a framework helps in the mutual interpretation of both speech and nonspeech data. Both types of movement are performed with the same set of BEPs, which doesn't necessarily mean that the neural control functions are identical. Nonspeech and speech functions can be related mutually with respect to their underlying BEPs. In this sense, measures such as maximal performance efforts (Kent, Kent, & Rosenbek, 1987) are relevant to an overall evaluation of the systems involved in speech production. However, the interpretation of data for tasks such as maximal performance efforts should consider the differential requirements of speech and nonspeech tasks. The interactions among functional units also are critical to a full assessment. For example, if one unit is dysfunctional in some way, is it likely that another interactive unit can compensate for the dysfunction? For another example, if several units are dysfunctional, is the total impairment due to their *combined* dysfunctions rather than what might be expected from their individual dysfunctions?

This framework helps the clinician or researcher to interpret the dysfunctions at various levels. That is, the framework is a means to assessment, or the interpretation of measurements. It is worth noting that speech-language pathology has a long history of quantitation, whether by perceptual scaling, behavioral inventories, or instrumental methods. Sometimes this quantitative orientation is forgotten in the history of this field. It is important to recall this orientation because the outlook for the future depends upon the agenda that is prepared for it. Some might argue that the field of motor speech disorders needs an infusion of quantitative methods, but this may not be the real problem.

In few clinical fields has quantitation been pursued with the same vigor as in speech-language pathology. For example, the classic neurologic examination has primary objectives that are not quantitative by their nature: 1) diagnose and localize a neurologic lesion, 2) identify the pathologic nature of the disorder, 3) estimate the prognosis, and 4) institute a therapeutic regimen. There is relatively little concern with objectively measuring the degree of neurologic impairment. Surely, there are neurologists and neuroscientists who promote quantitation. In the recent *Quantification of Neurologic Deficit*, Munsat (1989) reports on a workshop pertaining exactly to this issue. The preface contains this summary statement.

> Considerable discussion focused on whether quantitation beyond the classic neurologic examination would be acceptable or valuable to the average practicing neurologist. The consensus seemed to be that quantitation, as discussed in the workshop, would most likely remain the domain of the clinical researcher—at least for the near future. (p. ii)

Classic clinical examinations in speech-language pathology have a distinct quantitative flavor, even if attention is restricted to measures that can be made without specialized instrumentation. Speech-language pathologists inquire about the number of dysfluencies, severity of nasality, degree of hoarseness, rate of speaking in words per minute, habitual pitch level, diadochokinetic rate, duration of vowel phonation, rating of intelligibility, mean utterance length in morphemes, and so on. All these are quantitative. No apology need be made for using the senses of hearing, vision, and taction as means of gathering these kinds of data. The question, however, for the forward-looking clinician and scientist is: Can we do better by revising our perceptual methods, by incorporating instrumental techniques, and by shoring up those areas wherein there are shortcomings in validity, reliability, or even the means to make a relevant observation?

UNDERSTANDING SPEAKER VARIABLES AS THEY RELATE TO ISSUES IN ASSESSMENT AND MANAGEMENT

Issues in assessment and management have not been examined systematically in published research, and a research agendum could be constructed to address them. Speaker variables include age, sex, general cognitive status, physical health, and motivation. Many clinicians have a good understanding of these factors, but the research literature is rather weak and may not substantiate or facilitate clinical wisdom. Consider, for example, the simple question: Are males and females similar in the dysarthria associated with a given neurologic disorder? Unfortunately, the data are too limited to give a firm answer. However, recent research indicates that men and women have different profiles of impairment in the dysarthria associated with amyotrophic lateral sclerosis (Kent et al., 1992; Kent et al., 1990). Do similar male versus female differences occur in other forms of dysarthria? The answer to this question could be important for both clinical assessment and management.

In similar fashion, one might ask: How does dysarthria relate to a patient's age, cognitive status, and general physical condition? Unfortunately, not much is known in these areas, but the general literature on aging surely prompts attention to this factor. It is well documented that the physical structures and functions of speech undergo a number of changes with aging (Kent & Burkhard, 1981; Weismer & Liss, 1991). Moreover, some of these changes interact with speaker gender.

It seems that males may experience greater age-related loss of pulmonic and laryngeal function. Britt et al. (1981) reported data on gender differences in the age-related decline of pulmonary function. For nonsmoking men and women under the age of 45 years, the mean rates of decline were 16.7 and 22.0 ml/year, respectively. For nonsmoking subjects over 45 years of age, the rates were 42.8 ml/year for men and 27.7 ml/year for women. The rate of decline was about 65% greater for men. Although young, healthy men have about 10% more maximum aerobic power than young, healthy women (Boulay et al., 1984), aging effects are greater for males. The effects of smoking were roughly comparable for men and women. For smokers age 45 years or over, the rates of decline were 49.5 ml/year for men and 51.7 ml/year for women. It seems that the greatest risk for pulmonary decline is for male smokers. Laryngeal structure and function also are affected by aging, and the rates of senescent change are greater for men than for women (Weismer & Liss, 1991).

Gender-dependent changes in function with aging are of obvious relevance to the many speech motor disorders that tend to occur in older individuals, such as Parkinson's disease, amyotrophic lateral sclerosis, and stroke.

DEVELOPMENT AND EVALUATION OF MANAGEMENT STRATEGIES FOR DYSARTHRIA

More has been published on development than on evaluation. Although it is reassuring that management procedures have been described, relatively little effort has been given to evaluating their efficacy. Perhaps for the present, it is sufficient to know that a procedure works at all, let alone whether it is efficient, whether it is better than alternative approaches, or whether it is contraindicated by some patient characteristics. It is certainly a mark of progress that book-length coverage has been given to the management of motor speech disorders (Yorkston, Beukelman, & Bell, 1988) and that management figures more prominently in books for the current educational and professional markets than was the case just one or two decades ago. Substantial progress also has been made in augmentative and alternative communication (Beukelman & Mirenda, 1992).

Documenting change as the result of clinical intervention remains a concern. The use of single-subject designs has helped considerably, but even more fundamental issues need attention. One of these is measurement, particularly as it relates to standardization and efficiency. This topic is potentially vast, and only two examples are considered here. The first is an attempt to define an index of change. Tosi and Bertoccini (1990) proposed the following indices for changes in phonatory function, but they could easily be extended to other functional measures.

$$F = 100 \{1 - | (N - A) / (N - B) | \}$$
$$F = 100 \{[(N - |N - A|) - B] / N\}$$

where N = normal mean; B = individual subject's mean before treatment (or early in disease progression); A = individual subject's mean after treatment (or later stage in disease)

The second example comes from Bain and Dollaghan's (1991) development of an Intervention Efficiency Index (IEI).

IEI = Developmental Gain (months) / Time in Intervention (months)

Although this index is based on developmental gains in children, it would not be difficult to modify it to serve as an index of intervention efficiency for acquired disorders in adults, as:

IEI = Functional Gain / Time in Intervention

The functional gain could be measured in suitable units for the dimension(s) of interest, such as centimeters of water pressure for intraoral air pressure, time in seconds for vowel prolongation time, change in number of syllables per second for speaking rate determination, or decibels of sound pressure level (SPL) for vocal output.

Ideally, measures useful in assessment also will be useful in gauging the effects of intervention. Moreover, the same logic that enabled assessment can be used to develop, and revise as needed, a program of management.

CONCLUSION

Progress in research on dysarthria has not been uniform on all fronts of investigation. Certain core issues, such as taxonomy and nosology, remain relatively unexamined in the research literature, despite the fact that a good case can be made for further consideration of these issues. The greatest activity probably has been in the application and evaluation of a variety of methods to the laboratory study of dysarthria. Although these studies may not have altered greatly the understanding of pathophysiology, substantial progress has been made in the development and refinement of measurement procedures. Continued work may well result in breakthroughs in pathophysiology. It seems that increasing attention is being given to speaker variables as they relate to clinical assessment and management. However, the available published data on this topic are woefully inadequate to inform clinical practice. Finally, management of motor speech disorders is maturing, at least in terms of its presence in the literature.

REFERENCES

Adams, S.G. (1990). *Rate and clarity of speech: An x-ray microbeam study.* Unpublished doctoral dissertation, University of Wisconsin-Madison.

Arends, N., Povel, D.J., Van Os, E., & Speth, L. (1990). Predicting voice quality of deaf speakers on the basis of glottal characteristics. *Journal of Speech and Hearing Disorders, 29,* 156–170.

Bain, B., & Dollaghan, C. (1991). Treatment efficacy: The notion of clinically significant change. *Language, Speech and Hearing Services in Schools, 22,* 264–270.

Barlow, S.M. (1992). Recent advances in clinical speech physiology. In J. Cooper (Ed.), *Assessment of speech and voice production: Research and clinical applications,* NIDCD Monograph (pp. 183–195). Bethesda, MD: National Institute on Deafness and Other Communication Disorders.

Barlow, S.M., & Abbs, J.H. (1984). Orofacial fine motor control impairments in congenital spasticity: Evidence against hypertonus-related performance deficits. *Neurology, 34,* 145–150.

Beukelman, D.R., & Mirenda, P. (1992). *Augmentative and alternative communication: Management of severe communication disorders in children and adults.* Baltimore: Paul H. Brookes Publishing Co.

Boulay, M.R., Hamel, P., Simoneau, J.A., Lortie, G., Prud'homme, D., & Bouchard, C. (1984). A test of aerobic capacity: Description and reliability. *Canadian Journal of Applied Sport Science, 9,* 122–126.

Britt, E.J., Shelhamer, J., Menkes, H., Cohen, B., Meyer, M., & Permutt, S. (1981). Sex differences in the decline of pulmonary function with age. *Chest, 80* (Suppl.), 79S–80S.

Coleman, C.K., & Meyers, L.S. (1991). Computer recognition of the speech of adults with cerebral palsy and dysarthria. *Augmentative and Alternative Communication, 7,* 34–42.

Collins, M. (1984). Integrating perceptual and instrumental procedures in dysarthria assessment. *Communication Disorders, 5,* 159–170.

Darley, F.L., Aronson, A.E., & Brown, J.R. (1969a). Differential diagnostic patterns of dysarthria. *Journal of Speech and Hearing Research, 12,* 249–269.

Darley, F.L., Aronson, A.E., & Brown, J.R. (1969b). Cluster of deviant speech dimensions in the dysarthrias. *Journal of Speech and Hearing Research., 12,* 462–496.

Darley, F.L., Aronson, A.E., & Brown, J.R. (1975a). *Motor speech disorders.* Philadelphia: W.B. Saunders.

Darley, F.L., Aronson, A.E., & Brown, J.R. (1975b). *Audio seminars in speech pathology: Motor speech disorders.* Philadelphia: W.B. Saunders.

Eskenazi, L., Childers, D.G., & Hicks, D.M. (1990). Acoustic correlates of vocal quality. *Journal of Speech and Hearing Research, 33,* 298–306.

Gerratt, B.R., Till, J.A., Rosenbek, J.C., Wertz, R.T., & Boysen, A.E. (1991). Use and perceived value of perceptual and instrumental measures in dysarthria management. In C.A. Moore, K.M. Yorkston, & D.R. Beukelman (Eds.), *Dysarthria and apraxia of speech: Perspectives on management* (pp. 77–93). Baltimore: Paul H. Brookes Publishing Co.

Griffiths, C., & Bough, I.D., Jr. (1989). Neurologic diseases and their effect on voice. *Journal of Voice, 3,* 148–156.

Hicks, D.M. (1992). Functional voice assessment: What to measure and why. In J. Cooper (Ed.), *Assessment of voice and speech production: Research and clinical applications,* NIDCD Monograph (pp. 204–209). Bethesda, MD: National Institutes on Deafness and Other Communication Disorders.

Hillenbrand, J., & Flege, J.E. (1992). Application of acoustic techniques to the assessment of speech disorders. In J. Cooper (Ed.), *Assessment of speech and voice production: Research and clinical applications,* NIDCD Monograph (pp. 53–62). Bethesda, MD: National Institute on Deafness and Other Communication Disorders.

Kent, J.F., Kent, R.D., Rosenbeck, F.C., Weismer, G., Martin, R., Sufit, R., &

Brooks, B.R. (1992). Quantitative description of dysarthria in women with amyotrophic lateral sclerosis. *Journal of Speech and Hearing Research, 35,* 723–733.

Kent, R.D. (1992). Research needs in the assessment of speech motor disorders. In J. Cooper (Ed.), *Assessment of speech and voice production: Research and clinical applications,* NIDCD Monograph (Proceedings of a Conference, Sept. 27–28, 1990) (pp. 17–28). Bethesda, MD: National Institute on Deafness and other Communication Disorders.

Kent, R.D., & Burkhard, R. (1981). Changes in the acoustic correlates of speech production. In D.S. Beasley & G.A. Davis (Eds.), *Aging: Communication processes and disorders* (pp. 47–62). New York: Grune & Stratton.

Kent, R.D., Kent, J.F., & Rosenbek, J.C. (1987). Maximum performance tests of speech production. *Journal of Speech and Hearing Disorders, 52,* 367–387.

Kent, R.D., Kent, J.F., Weismer, G., Sufit, R.L, Rosenbek, J.C., Martin, R.E., & Brooks, B.R. (1990). Impairment of speech intelligibility in men with amyotrophic lateral sclerosis. *Journal of Speech and Hearing Disorders, 55,* 721–728.

Kent, R.D., & Netsell, R. (1978) Articulatory abnormalities in athetoid cerebral palsy. *Journal of Speech and Hearing Disorders, 43,* 353–373.

Kent, R.D., Weismer, G., Kent, J.F., & Rosenbek, J.C. (1989). Toward phonetic intelligibility testing in dysarthria. *Journal of Speech and Hearing Disorders, 54,* 482–499.

Kondraske, G.V. (1989). Measurement science concepts and computerized methodology in the assessment of human performance. In T.L. Munsat (Ed.), *Quantification of neurologic deficit* (pp. 33–48). Boston: Butterworths.

Kreiman, J., Gerratt, B.R., & Precoda, K. (1990). Listener experience and perception of voice quality. *Journal of Speech and Hearing Research, 33,* 103–115.

Kreiman, J., Gerratt, B.R., Precoda, K., & Berke, G.S. (1992). Individual differences in voice quality perception. *Journal of Speech and Hearing Research, 35,* 512–520.

Lance, J.W. (1980). Symposium synopsis. In R.G. Feldman, R.R. Young, & W.P. Keollo (Eds.), *Spasticity: Disordered motor control* (pp. 485–494). Chicago: Yearbook Medical Publishers.

Muller, E.M., & Brown, W.S. (1980). Variations in the supraglottal air pressure waveform and their articulatory interpretations. In N.J. Lass (Ed.), *Speech and language: Advances in basic research and practice* (Vol. 4, pp. 317–389). New York: Academic Press.

Munsat, T.L. (Ed.). (1989). *Quantification of neurologic deficit.* Boston: Butterworths.

Myklebust, B.M., Gottlieb, G.L., Penn, R.D., & Agarwal, G.C. (1982). Reciprocal excitation of antagonistic muscles as a differentiating feature in spasticity. *Annals of Neurology, 12,* 367–374.

Neilson, P.D., & O'Dwyer, N.J. (1981). Pathophysiology of dysarthria in cerebral palsy. *Journal of Neurology, Neurosurgery and Psychiatry, 44,* 1013–1019.

Netsell, R.W. (1986). *A neurobiologic view of speech production and the dysarthrias.* San Diego: College-Hill.

Orlikoff, R.F. (in press). The use of instrumental measures in the assessment and treatment of motor speech disorders. *Seminars in Speech and Language.*

Putnam, A.H.B. (1988). Review of research in dysarthria. In H. Winitz (Ed.), *Human communication and its disorders* (Vol. 2, pp. 107–223). Norwood, NJ: Ablex.

Rosenbek, J.C., & McNeil, M.R. (1991). A discussion of classification in motor speech disorders: Dysarthria and apraxia of speech. In C.A. Moore, K.M. Yorkston, & D.R. Beukelman (Eds.), *Dysarthria and apraxia of speech: Perspectives on management* (pp. 289–295). Baltimore: Paul H. Brookes Publishing Co.

Schiavetti, N. (1992). Scaling procedures for the measurement of speech intelligibility. In R.D. Kent (Ed.), *Intelligibility in speech disorders: Theory, measurement, and management* (pp. 11–34). Philadelphia: John Benjamins North America.

Seikel, J.A., Wilcox, K.A., & Davis, J. (1990). Dysarthria of motor neuron disease: Clinician judgments of severity. *Journal of Communication Disorders, 23,* 417–431.

Sheard, C., Adams, R.D., & Davis, P.J. (1991). Reliability and agreement of ratings of ataxic dysarthric speech samples with varying intelligibility. *Journal of Speech and Hearing Research, 34,* 285–293.

Southwood, H. (1990). *Bizarreness, acceptability, naturalness, and normalcy of speech of ALS speakers.* Unpublished doctoral dissertation, University of Wisconsin-Madison.

Till, J.A., & Alp, L.A. (1991). Aerodynamic and temporal measures of continuous speech in dysarthric speakers. In C.A. Moore, K.M. Yorkston, & D.R. Beukelman (Eds.), *Dysarthria and apraxia of speech: Perspectives on management* (pp. 185–203). Baltimore: Paul H. Brookes Publishing Co.

Tosi, O., & Bertoccini, G. (1990). Phoniatric indices of change. *Folia Phoniatrica, 42,* 150–152.

Warren, D.W. (1992). Aerodynamic measurements of speech. In J. Cooper (Ed.), *Assessment of speech and voice production: Research and clinical applications,* NIDCD Monograph (pp. 103–111). Bethesda, MD: National Institute on Deafness and Other Communication Disorders.

Weismer, G., & Liss, J.M. (1991). Age and speech motor control. In D. Ripich (Ed.), *Handbook of aging and communication* (pp. 205–226). Austin, TX: PRO-ED.

Weismer, G., & Martin, R.E. (1992). Acoustic and perceptual approaches to the study of intelligibility. In R.D. Kent (Ed.), *Intelligibility in speech disorders: Theory, measurement and management* (pp. 68–118). Philadelphia: John Benjamins North America.

Wolf, V.I., & Steinfatt, T.M. (1987). Prediction of vocal severity within and across voice types. *Journal of Speech and Hearing Research, 30,* 230–240.

Yorkston, K., & Beukelman, D.R. (1981). Communication efficiency of dysarthric speakers as measured by sentence intelligibility and speaking rate. *Journal of Speech and Hearing Disorders, 46,* 296–301.

Yorkston, K.M., Beukelman, D.R., & Bell, K.R. (1988). *Clinical management of dysarthric speakers.* Boston: College-Hill.

Ziegler, W. (1991, March 25–26). *Acoustic and perceptual methods in the clinical evaluation of dysarthric speech.* Paper presented at the 1st Symposium of the International Clinical Phonetics and Linguistics Association, Advances in Clinical Phonetics, Cardiff Institute of Higher Education, Cardiff, Wales, U.K.

Ziegler, W., Hartmann, E., & von Cramon, D. (1988). Word identification testing in the diagnostic evaluation of dysarthric speech. *Clinical Linguistics and Phonetics, 2,* 291–308.

Zwirner, P., Murry, T., & Woodson, G.E. (1991). Phonatory function of neurologically impaired patients. *Journal of Communication Disorders, 24,* 287–300.

Zyski, B.J., & Weisiger, B.E. (1987). Identification of dysarthria types based on perceptual analysis. *Journal of Communication Disorders, 20,* 367–378.

Chapter 2

Dysarthria from the Viewpoint of Individuals with Dysarthria

Kathryn M. Yorkston,
Charles Bombardier, and Vicki L. Hammen

DYSARTHRIA, AS EVERY complex phenomenon, may be viewed from many different perspectives. The neurologist may see dysarthria as a symptom of neurologic disease. The speech physiologist may see it as a means of understanding contributors to speech production. The speech-language pathologist may see it as a disability to remediate. All these perspectives have received considerable attention in the literature. Perhaps the most neglected perspective on dysarthria is that of the individual with dysarthria. With a few notable exceptions (Berry, Evans, & Lane, 1990; Berry, & Sanders, 1983; Gies-Zaborowski & Silverman, 1986), we have not examined dysarthria from the point of view of the speaker with dysarthria. This chapter is a preliminary investigation of how individuals with dysarthria experience their disability. Our questions are do speakers with mild, moderate, and severe dysarthria differ in: 1) the number of speech characteristics they endorse, 2) the number and types of communication situations they find difficult, 3) the compensatory strategies they find to be beneficial, and 4) the perceived reactions of others to their dysarthria?

This work was supported in part by Grant #H133B80081 from the National Institute on Disability and Rehabilitation Research, Department of Education, Washington, D.C. This work is in the public domain. We thank Dave Beukelman and Marsha Sullivan, University of Nebraska, for their assistance in soliciting subjects.

19

METHODS

Questionnaire

A 100-item questionnaire (the appendix to this chapter) was developed to solicit information in the following areas: characteristics of the disorder, situational difficulty, compensatory strategies, and perceived reactions of others. The initial pool of items was generated from a number of sources including a review of questionnaires designed to assess the degree of disability associated with hearing impairment (Demorest & Erdman, 1986, 1987; Demorest & Walden, 1984), interviews with individuals with dysarthria, and suggestions from speech-language pathologists.

Characteristics Thirteen items were developed in order to obtain information about the speaker's perception of the features of the dysarthria. For example, "My speech is slow," "My speech is difficult for strangers to understand," and "My voice sounds hoarse or harsh."

Situational Difficulty In the initial phase of this project, our goal was to create a series of items that represented a broad range of difficulty, while at the same time included situations typically encountered by most adults with dysarthria. After the initial pool of items had been developed, seven speech-language pathologists were asked to rate each situation according to six dimensions that were assumed to influence ease of communication. These dimensions were: partner familiarity (PF), size of audience (SA), demand for intelligibility (DI), demand for speed (DS), emotional load (EL), and environmental adversity (EA). Table 1 contains the rating scales used for each characteristic, the number of items receiving an average score of two or higher across raters, and examples of items rated high for each dimension. Judges' responses were used to eliminate confusing items, items on which judges disagreed, or items not generally applicable to an adult population. Cumulative difficulty scores ranged from zero ("telling a family member what you would like for breakfast" was not considered difficult on any of the situational dimensions) to six ("asking for information in a group or class" was considered difficult on all six dimensions).

Compensatory Strategies Potential strategies or techniques for handling difficult communication situations were also developed. A panel of speech-language pathologists was asked to place each strategy into one of the following categories: 1) *Improved production*—items in this category suggest that speakers attempt to improve speech production; for example, "If someone has misunderstood part of what I have said, I repeat the message more clearly"; 2) *Environmental modification*—items in this category suggest that speakers eliminate unfavorable environmental characteristics; for example, "When I am involved in an important conversation, I turn off the radio, TV, or other noise sources"; 3) *Avoidance*—items in

Table 1. Ratings of situational difficulty

Domains	Rating scale	Number of items receiving high scores[a]	Examples of items receiving high scores
Partner familiarity (PF)	0—Not applicable 1—Very familiar 2—Familiar 3—Unfamiliar	8	At a restaurant ordering food or drinks Asking a bus driver for directions
Size of audience (SA)	0—Not applicable 1—One-on-one 2—Small 3—Large	5	Asking for information in a group or class At a dinner party with several other people
Demand for intelligibility (DI)	0—Not applicable 1—Low 2—Medium 3—High	24	Talking with my doctor about a medical problem Upset and trying to get a point across
Demand for speed (DS)	0—Not applicable 1—Low 2—Medium 3—High	19	At a meeting with several other people Explaining to a friend that something exciting has happened
Emotional load (EL)	0—Not applicable 1—Low 2—Medium 3—High	15	Trying to resolve a conflict with someone Making a difficult request of someone
Environmental adversity (EA)	0—Not applicable 1—Low 2—Medium 3—High	12	Chatting with someone while riding in a car Having a conversation at a social gathering while others are nearby, the room is dimly lit

[a]A high score is defined as an average score of two or higher across judges.

this category suggest that speakers avoid potentially difficult situations; for example, "I tend to be merely a listener in conversations so I won't have to speak"; 4) *Message modification*—items in this category suggest that speakers change the message or mode of communication in response to potentially difficult situations; for example, "If someone has misunderstood me, I use different wording when I repeat the message"; 5) *Partner instruction*—items in this category suggest that speakers give directions to their communication partners; for example, "When people have trouble understanding me, I ask them to watch me as I speak." Thirty items were selected for which there was high interjudge agreement.

   Perceived Reactions of Others   Items describing the reactions of others to the dysarthria were drawn from Kerns, Turk, and Rudy (1985). Seven speech-language pathologists were asked to place each item into one of the following categories: 1) *Helpful*—items in this category suggest a constructive or beneficial response by communication partners; for example, "People encourage me to speak for myself"; 2) *Solicitous*—items in this category suggest excessive concern for the speaker's welfare; for example, "Others order for me in a restaurant, although I would prefer to do it myself"; and 3) *Punishing*—items in this category suggest that others are penalizing the speaker with dysarthria; for example, "Because of my speech problem, people treat me as if I am not very bright."

Description of Speakers with Dysarthria

Table 2 contains information about the 33 adults with dysarthria who participated in this study. Note that 10 subjects exhibited mild dysarthria (sentence production is intelligible), 16 exhibited moderate dysarthria (sentence intelligibility between 50% and 95%), and 7 had severe dysarthria (sentence intelligibility less than 50%), but all subjects used natural speech as the sole means of communication. Medical diagnoses included amyotrophic lateral sclerosis ($N = 12$), Parkinson's disease ($N = 7$), traumatic brain injury ($N = 6$), cerebral palsy ($N = 2$), and other ($N = 4$). Subjects ranged in age from 18 to 80 years with a mean age of 62.8 and a standard deviation of 21.8 years. The group included 15 males and 18 females. All subjects had experienced symptoms of dysarthria for at least three months. Note that for a number of the subjects with amyotrophic lateral sclerosis (ALS) dysarthria symptoms preceded diagnosis.

RESULTS

Item Analysis

Removal of "Not Applicable" Items Recall that our goal was to include a range of item difficulty, and in addition, to include items commonly applicable across subjects with dysarthria. Therefore, our first analysis was to calculate the proportion of subjects who indicated that an item was "not applicable" to them. Three of the 30 situational difficulty items were considered not applicable by more than 30% of subjects. These items all pertained to employment. (You are explaining a new project to someone at work; You are talking on the telephone with a new client; and You are talking to a co-worker in an office.) Because of the difficulty of interpreting results from items for which there is a high percentage of "not applicable" responses, these three items were excluded from the analysis and the analysis was performed on the remaining 27 items.

Distribution of Difficulty Scores The percentage of subjects endorsing each item in the areas of speech characteristics, situational difficulty, compensatory strategies, and perceived reactions of others was calculated. Items in each area were rank ordered from least to most frequently endorsed. These data are shown in Figure 1 A–D. Note that the percentage of subjects endorsing each item ranged from approximately 20% to approximately 80%. Thus, items were always endorsed by at least some subjects, but no items were endorsed by all subjects.

Speech Characteristics Endorsed

Our first question was: Do speakers with mild, moderate, and severe dysarthria differ in the number of speech characteristics they endorse? Figure 2 illustrates the mean proportion of speech characteristics endorsed for the groups with mild, moderate, and severe dysarthria. Although the mean scores for the severe group were slightly higher than the others, a one-way analysis of variance indicated that the differences were not statistically significant ($p = .304$). Thus, speakers with mild, moderate, and severe dysarthria in this study did not differ in the number of speech characteristics they endorsed.

Situational Difficulty

The next question was: Do speakers with dysarthria of varying severities differ in the number and types of communication situations they find difficult? In order to answer this, responses to items that were rated difficult on each of the situational domains were examined for each severity group. Results of that analysis are illustrated in Figure 3, which contains plots of proportion of items in each domain that were endorsed as difficult by the mild, moderate, and severely involved groups. Note that the severely involved group tended to endorse more items as difficult. However, a two-way analysis of variance was performed with no significant main effects for severity group, situational dimensions, and no significant group by situation interaction (see Table 3). Thus, speakers with mild, moderate, and severe dysarthria did not differ in the number or types of communication situations they found difficult.

Compensatory Strategies

Our third question was: Do speakers with dysarthria of varying severities differ in the compensatory strategies they find to be beneficial? Figure 4 illustrates the mean percentage of strategies endorsed by groups with mild, moderate, and severe dysarthria. The strategies include improved production, avoidance, environmental modification, message modification, and partner instruction. A two-way analysis of variance (see Table 4) revealed no main effect for severity group although the group with severe dysarthria tended to endorse environmental and message modification more than the other groups. The effect for strategy was significant with post hoc analysis indicating the strategy of improved production was endorsed more frequently than others. No interaction between severity and compensatory strategy was found. Thus, the speakers with mild, moderate,

Table 2. Characteristics of subjects

Subject number	Severity of dysarthria	Medical diagnosis	Age/ gender	Months post-onset	Employment status
1	Mild	Parkinson's disease	75/M	48	Retired
2	Mild	Amyotrophic lateral sclerosis	74/F	2[a]	Retired
3	Mild	Amyotrophic lateral sclerosis	53/F	4[a]	Retired
4	Mild	Amyotrophic lateral sclerosis	64/M	8[a]	Retired
5	Mild	Cerebral vascular accident	64/M	3	Retired
6	Mild	Amyotrophic lateral sclerosis	63/M	1[a]	Retired
7	Mild	Amyotrophic lateral sclerosis	64/F	2[a]	Retired
8	Mild	Amyotrophic lateral sclerosis	55/F	20[a]	Retired
9	Mild	Parkinson's disease	57/M	180	Retired
10	Mild	Cerebral vascular accident	54/F	4	Restaurant manager
11	Moderate	Amyotrophic lateral sclerosis	64/M	20[a]	Contractor
12	Moderate	Acoustic neuroma	33/M	45	Volunteer work
13	Moderate	Traumatic brain injury	19/F	37	Student
14	Moderate	Traumatic brain injury	35/F	112	Homemaker
15	Moderate	Amyotrophic lateral sclerosis	62/M	16	Retired
16	Moderate	Multiple sclerosis	48/M	120	Engineer

	Severity	Diagnosis	Age/Sex	Months	Occupation
17	Moderate	Traumatic brain injury	24/M	30	Unemployed
18	Moderate	Parkinson's disease	77/M	60	Retired
19	Moderate	Parkinson's disease	55/M	60	Management analyst
20	Moderate	Parkinson's disease	58/F	60	Retired
21	Moderate	Parkinson's disease	75/M	180	Retired
22	Moderate	Parkinson's disease	70/M	36	Salesman
23	Moderate	Cerebellar degeneration	41/F	156	Unemployed
24	Moderate	Amyotrophic lateral sclerosis	80/F	8[a]	Unemployed
25	Moderate	Amyotrophic lateral sclerosis	63/F	6	Retired
26	Moderate	Amyotrophic lateral sclerosis	41/F	2[a]	Sales associate
27	Severe	Amyotrophic lateral sclerosis	67/F	2[a]	Retired
28	Severe	Traumatic brain injury	30/M	8	Unemployed
29	Severe	Cerebral palsy	44/F	congenital	Volunteer work
30	Severe	Cerebral palsy	61/F	congenital	Homemaker
31	Severe	Traumatic brain injury	23/F	18	Unemployed
32	Severe	Traumatic brain injury	42/F	96	Unemployed
33	Severe	Anoxia	18/F	15	Student

[a]Months post-diagnosis of ALS.

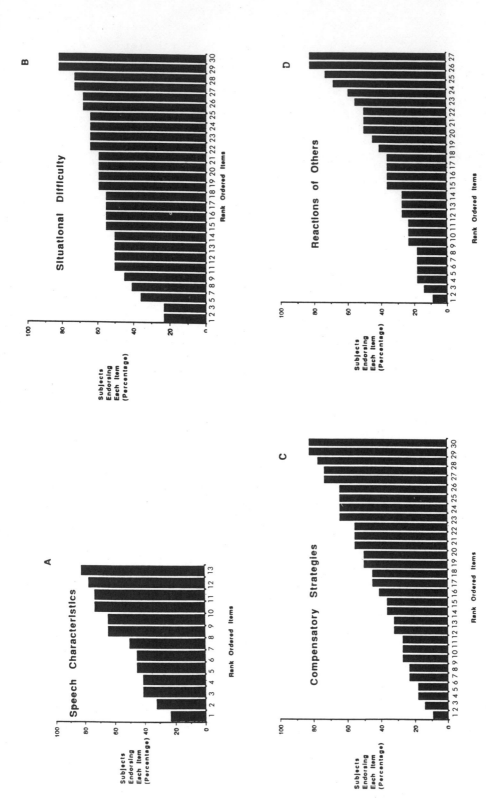

Figure 1. Percentage of subjects endorsing each item in the areas of: (A) speech characteristics, (B) situational difficulty, (C) compensatory strategies, and (D) reactions of others. Items are rank ordered from those least frequently endorsed to those most frequently endorsed.

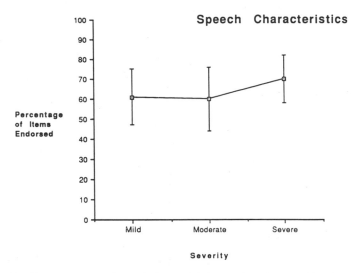

Figure 2. Mean percentage of speech characteristic items endorsed across subjects in groups with mild, moderate, and severe dysarthria. Also noted are standard deviation bars.

and severe dysarthria did not differ in the number or type of compensatory strategies they found to be beneficial. All subjects felt that improved production was the most beneficial strategy. We return later to a discussion of the single strategy of "improved production" that was endorsed so frequently.

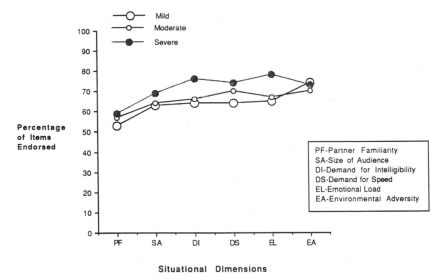

Figure 3. Mean percentage of items endorsed for each situational dimension for groups with mild, moderate, and severe dysarthria.

Table 3. Analysis of variance for the factors severity of dysarthria and situational difficulty

Source	Sum of squares	df	Mean square	F-ratio	p
Severity	1537.15	2	768.57	1.38	.254
Situational difficulty	4764.86	5	952.97	1.71	.134
Severity by situational difficulty	814.93	10	81.49	0.15	.999

Perceived Reactions of Others

Our final question was: Do speakers with dysarthria of varying severities differ in how they perceive reactions of others to their dysarthria? Responses to items related to reactions of others were categorized as helpful, solicitous, or punishing, and the mean percentages of items endorsed were computed for the groups with mild, moderate, and severe dysarthria. Figure 5 illustrates the results of this analysis. Note that items categorized as helpful were endorsed most frequently, whereas items categorized as punishing were endorsed least frequently. Also note that, in general, the subjects with severe dysarthria endorsed more items. The main effects of severity groups and type of reactions were significant (Table 5). The inter-

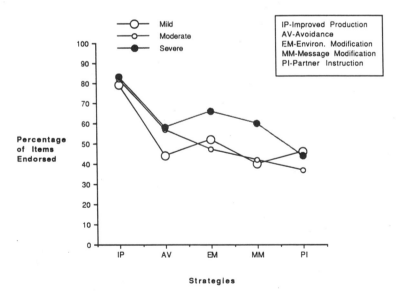

Figure 4. Mean percentage of items endorsed for each category of compensatory strategy for groups with mild, moderate, and severe dysarthria.

Table 4. Analysis of variance for the factors severity of dysarthria and compensatory strategy

Source	Sum of squares	df	Mean square	F-ratio	p
Severity	2400.53	2	1200.27	1.74	.179
Compensatory strategy	26765.58	4	6691.39	9.69	.000
Severity by compensatory strategy	3063.6	8	382.95	0.55	.814

action of severity by type of reaction was nonsignificant. Thus, individuals with severe dysarthria differ from others in their perception of the reactions of others to their dysarthria. Generally, individuals with severe dysarthria felt that others were more helpful, more solicitous, and more punishing than did individuals with less severe dysarthria.

DISCUSSION

A number of directions for future research have resulted from this work. We were somewhat surprised by the lack of differences among the severity groups for number of speech characteristics endorsed, type and frequency of situations felt to be difficult, and the number of compensatory strategies found to be beneficial. The clearest distinction between the severity groups was found in the area of perceived reactions of others. This suggests that asking questions about perceived reactions of others may be a

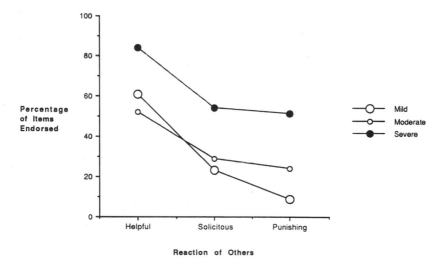

Figure 5. Mean percentage of items endorsed for each category of reactions of others for groups with mild, moderate, and severe dysarthria.

Table 5. Analysis of variance for the factors severity of dysarthria and perceived reactions of others

Source	Sum of squares	df	Mean square	F-ratio	p
Severity	14676.18	2	7338.09	15.356	.000
Perceived reactions	23831.48	2	11915.74	24.94	.000
Severity by perceived reactions	1945.12	4	486.3	1.02	.403

reasonable means of assessing the degree of handicap associated with dysarthria. Much attention has been given to the development of satisfactory physiologic tools to measure the impairment in dysarthria. Likewise, attention has been given to the development of perceptual tools, such as intelligibility ratings, to measure the disability associated with dysarthria. The data reported here point us in the direction of better measurement of handicap.

The second direction of future research is the investigation of differences among diagnostic groups. Recall that our subject groups were categorized by severity of dysarthria rather than by medical diagnosis. As we began to accumulate responses from many individuals with dysarthria, we began to consider the possibility that diagnosis category was also an important dimension to consider, because individuals with differing medical etiologies may respond differently. The following remarks are illustrated with some data from the parkinsonian sample. Figure 6 illustrates group data from the situational difficulty portion of the questionnaire and data from two individuals with Parkinson's disease. On the top is a parkinsonian speaker with speech that is over 95% intelligible, yet this individual endorses more situations as difficult than subjects in the group with severe dysarthria. On the other hand, the individual with Parkinson's disease and more severe dysarthria (lower portion of the figure) found almost nothing to be difficult. An explanation of these responses may be that some parkinsonian speakers do not have a proper appreciation of the extent of their disability. Future work will involve comparing severity-matched groups of parkinsonian and patients with ALS to examine the differences between diagnostic categories.

The final direction for this type of work is to document the impact of intervention. This can be examined by comparing the relative number of situations felt to be difficult before and after treatment. Figure 7 illustrates the responses of two individuals who are not functional communicators when they use natural speech. They completed our questionnaire after they had acquired and learned to use speech output augmentative communication systems. Generally, they reported that relatively few communication situations were difficult.

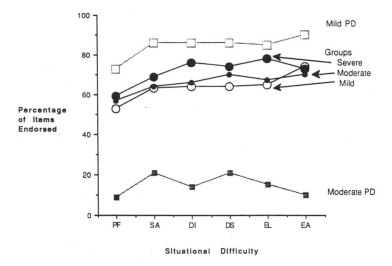

Figure 6. Mean percentage of items endorsed for each situational dimension for a parkinsonian speaker with mild dysarthria (Mild PD) and a parkinsonian speaker with moderate dysarthria (Moderate PD). Also presented for comparison are the mean responses of groups with mild, moderate, and severe dysarthria.

Other types of intervention might also be documented via the questionnaire. Recall that improved production was endorsed as the most effective strategy for all speakers with dysarthria, regardless of degree of severity. All other strategies were endorsed less frequently. This finding

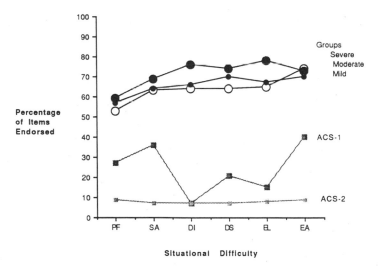

Figure 7. Mean percentage of items endorsed for each situational dimension for two users of augmentative communication systems (ACS-1 and ACS-2). Also presented for comparison are the mean responses of groups with mild, moderate, and severe dysarthria.

could be interpreted in at least two ways. On one hand, improved production may be the most effective technique for all speakers with dysarthria. On the other hand, our results may reflect our lack of emphasis in speech treatment on pragmatic aspects of communication; that is, use of compensatory strategies such as environmental manipulation and partner instruction. Questionnaires such as the one described in this chapter may prove to be reasonable avenues for documenting a changing use of compensatory strategies as a result of pragmatically based intervention.

REFERENCES

Berry, W., Evans, Y., & Lane, A. (1990). *The importance of patient attitude variables in dysarthria rehabilitation.* Paper presented at the Clinical Dysarthria Conference, San Antonio.

Berry, W., & Sanders, S. (1983). Environmental education: The universal management approach for adults with dysarthria. In W. Berry (Ed.), *Clinical dysarthria.* Boston: College-Hill.

Demorest, M.E., & Erdman, S.A. (1986). Scale composition and item analysis of the communication profile for the hearing impaired. *Journal of Speech and Hearing Research, 29,* 515–535.

Demorest, M.E., & Erdman, S.A. (1987). Development of the communication profile for the hearing impaired. *Journal of Speech and Hearing Disorders, 52,* 129–143.

Demorest, M.E., & Walden, B.E. (1984). Psychometric principles in the selection, interpretation, and evaluation of communication self-assessment inventories. *Journal of Speech and Hearing Disorders, 49,* 226–240.

Gies-Zaborowski, J., & Silverman, F. (1986). Documenting the impact of a mild dysarthria on peer perception. *Language, Speech and Hearing Services in Schools, 17,* 143.

Kerns, R., Turk, D., & Rudy, T. (1985). The West Haven–Yale multidimensional pain inventory (WHYMPI). *Pain, 23,* 345–356.

Appendix A

Questionnaire Items

Characteristics

1. My speech will improve if I work hard.
2. I can usually make strangers feel at ease with me.
3. I am skilled at handling difficult speaking situations.
4. My speech is difficult for strangers to understand.
5. My speech problem is so severe that it is difficult for my family to understand.
6. My speech is slow.
7. My speech is sometimes too loud or too soft.
8. I have difficulty speaking when I am in a hurry.
9. My speaking is poorer when I am tired.
10. My speech sounds unnatural.
11. My voice sounds hoarse or harsh.
12. My speech is going to improve.
13. My speech has a nasal quality.

Situational Difficulty

1. You are chatting with someone while riding in a car.
2. You are at a social gathering with friends, music is playing in the background, and someone starts a casual conversation.
3. You are talking with your family after dinner.
4. You are explaining a new project to someone at work.
5. You are at a restaurant ordering food or drinks.
6. You are talking on the telephone with a new client.
7. You are attempting to convey important information over the telephone in an emergency.
8. You are talking to someone in your family while you are watching TV or listening to the radio.
9. You are asking for information in a group or class.
10. You are talking to a co-worker in an office.
11. You are in a quiet room at home talking on the telephone.
12. You are at a dinner party with several other people.
13. You are speaking with someone who is obviously in a hurry.
14. You are at a meeting with several other people.
15. You are at home and you are talking to someone in another room.
16. You are having a conversation at a social gathering while others are talking nearby, the room is dimly lit.

Situational Difficulty
(continued)

17. You are talking with a friend or family member in a quiet room.
18. You are talking with your doctor about a medical problem.
19. You are trying to resolve a billing problem with a clerk.
20. You are asking a bus driver for directions.
21. You are talking with a close friend about emotional issues.
22. You are upset and trying to get a point across.
23. You are trying to resolve a conflict with someone.
24. You are making a difficult request of someone.
25. You are explaining to a friend that something exciting has happened.
26. You are angry and you want to let someone know it.
27. You are greeting an old friend.
28. You are telling a family member what you would like for breakfast.
29. You are trying to get the attention of someone in another room.
30. You are giving a formal presentation to a group.

Compensatory Strategies

1. I let my family or friends "translate" because I hate to repeat when strangers don't understand.
2. At parties or other social gatherings I try to stay in a well-lighted area so people can see me.
3. If someone has misunderstood part of what I have said, I repeat the message more clearly.
4. I let people know the topic of the message at the beginning of the conversation.
5. I don't change topics without letting my listener know.
6. I tell others to signal me when they are having difficulty understanding.
7. I make sure that people face me when I am speaking to them.
8. If someone seems irritated when they cannot understand me, I give up.
9. I avoid talking to strangers because of my speech problems.
10. When I am involved in an important conversation, I turn off the radio, TV, or other noise sources.
11. If my listener does not understand, then I try to repeat more clearly.
12. I speak louder when people have difficulty understanding me.
13. I stop frequently to let people ask me questions about what I have said.
14. I ask people to repeat what I have said to them so that I know they have understood.
15. I get people's attention before trying to communicate with them.
16. I always watch the listeners so I can tell when they do not understand me.
17. I tend to be merely a listener in conversations so I won't have to speak.
18. In difficult speaking situations, I try to position myself so that I can be seen when I am talking.
19. I try to speak more precisely when people are having difficulty understanding me.
20. If someone has misunderstood part of what I have said, I will write or spell out the message.
21. If someone has misunderstood me, I use different wording when I repeat the message.
22. I tell people not to interrupt until I am finished.
23. I ask people to be patient when talking with me.

24. I tend to avoid situations when I think I will have trouble being understood.
25. If people are not watching me as I speak, I move so that they can see me.
26. I avoid trying to talk with someone at a distance or someone in the next room.
27. I speak more slowly when people have difficulty understanding me.
28. When people have trouble understanding me, I ask them to watch me as I speak.
29. When I first meet strangers I try to let them know about my speech problem.
30. I signal to my listeners when I want a turn in the conversation.

Perceived Reactions of Others

1. People remind me to slow down or look at them when I speak.
2. People work hard to make communication easy for me.
3. Because of my speech problem, people treat me as if I am not very bright.
4. Others get irritated with my speech.
5. Others ignore me if they do not understand what I am saying.
6. Others treat me like a child when it comes to communication.
7. Others have taken over making telephone calls for me.
8. People tend to get impatient because I speak slowly.
9. Others praise me when I try to speak for myself.
10. Others interrupt me when they are having difficulty understanding me.
11. People treat me as if I can't do the job when I know that I am able.
12. People fill in words for me before I have a chance to complete my thought.
13. Others order for me in a restaurant, although I would prefer to do it myself.
14. Others criticize me for the way I talk.
15. People include me in conversation despite my speech problem.
16. Members of my family let me know when they do not understand me.
17. People paraphrase what I say to let me know that they understand me.
18. My family is patient when trying to communicate with me.
19. People leave me out of conversations.
20. People treat me as if I am hard of hearing.
21. People speak louder when talking to me because they think I have a hearing problem.
22. Family or friends tell me to not work so hard trying to speak.
23. Others have taken over my responsibilities because of my speech problem.
24. Others laugh or joke about my speech problem.
25. People encourage me to speak for myself.
26. When I am talking, people pretend to understand.
27. Others say they will speak for me whenever I want them to do so.

Chapter 3

Description and Classification of Individuals with Dysarthria
A 10-Year Review

Edythe A. Strand and Kathryn M. Yorkston

AS THE STUDY of dysarthria matures, clinical researchers must continue to search for new and better methods of investigation. Discussion at clinical dysarthria conferences has focused on these important issues: 1) the need to develop and use standard measurement tools and protocols for assessing and describing dysarthric speech, 2) the need to select appropriate levels of analysis, 3) the need for more investigations based on conceptual models of speech production, and 4) the need for critical evaluation of existing taxonomies with the goal of developing more useful classification systems. Central to all these issues are methods of speaker description and classification. Of particular interest to the authors is the need to determine the extent to which uniform practices of such description and classification are used in the clinical dysarthria literature. This chapter summarizes the results of a literature review designed with the following purposes in mind.

1. To examine subject description practices
2. To examine the criteria used for selecting and grouping subjects for a specific research question

This work was supported in part by Grant No. H133B80081 from the National Institute on Disability and Rehabilitation Research, Department of Education, Washington, D.C.
This work was also supported in part by Grant No. 1K08 DC00043-01A1 from NIDCD, National Institutes of Health. This work is in the public domain.

3. To discuss how procedures for selecting and grouping subjects are related to current taxonomies used in dysarthria research
4. To discuss the clinical and research implications of these current practices

METHODS

Manuscripts Reviewed

Manuscripts reporting data related to dysarthria published from 1982 through 1991 were reviewed. A standard form was used to record general information about each study and to tally and describe subject variables reported. Eighty-six manuscripts were identified through computerized library searches and volume-by-volume perusal of journals expected to contain articles related to dysarthria. (See Appendix A for complete list of manuscripts.)

Forty-five articles were identified from seven journals (Table 1). In addition, edited books representing a dense source of manuscripts related to dysarthria were included and increased the number of manuscripts reviewed to 86. Of the 86 manuscripts, 60 reported group data and 26 reported data regarding individual cases. Although both case presentations and group studies were included, only manuscripts that contained original data were reviewed. Thus, review articles or manuscripts containing only summaries of data published elsewhere were not included. A total of 774 subjects were included in the 86 manuscripts, although it was apparent that, at times, the same subjects were used in more than one article.

In order to determine whether interest in dysarthria (as measured by numbers of published manuscripts) has been constant over the last 10 years, and whether or not such interest may be increasing, the number of manuscripts reporting dysarthria data per year was totaled. Figure 1 illustrates the considerable variability from year to year in number of articles published. This variability is due primarily to the edited books on dysarthria that were published in 1983, 1984, 1989, and 1991. It is interesting to note that from 1982 through 1991, there were six or fewer manuscripts relating to dysarthria published in journals per year, except for 1990, during which 10 such manuscripts were published.

Descriptors of Individuals with Dysarthria

A list of 18 categories of descriptors was developed to reflect a broad range of the type of information that might be of interest when presenting the characteristics of a dysarthric sample (Table 2). As each manuscript was

Table 1. Manuscript sources for the group and case studies reviewed

Source	Group studies	Case studies	Total
Journals			
Journal of the Acoustical Society of America	4	0	4
Brain and Language	3	0	3
British Journal of Disorders of Communication	4	3	7
Folia Phoniatrica	2	1	3
Journal of Communication Disorders	7	3	10
Journal of Speech and Hearing Disorders	6	2	8
Journal of Speech and Hearing Research	8	2	10
Books[a]	26	15	41
Total	60	26	86

[a]See Appendix A.

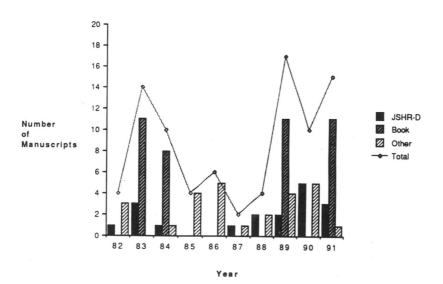

Figure 1. Number of manuscripts reporting dysarthria data per year. *Journal of Speech and Hearing Research* (JSHR) and *Journal of Speech and Hearing Disorders* (JSHD) are noted in the black bars. Edited books are indicated by the dark diagonal lines. The other journals are shown with the light diagonal lines. The line graph illustrates the total per year.

Table 2. Categories of subject descriptors used in manuscripts[a]

Medical diagnosis	Cognition and language
Age	Neurologic exam data
Sex	Severity of dysarthria
Disease severity	Medications
Time post-onset	Treatment history
Type of dysarthria	Hearing and vision
Physiologic data	Diadochokineses
Speech characteristics	Socioeconomic status and education
	Sensation
Acoustic data	

[a]Descriptors are listed in rank order of frequency of occurrence, rather than alphabetically (see Figure 2).

reviewed, a decision was made regarding the presence or absence of each descriptor anywhere in that manuscript. Furthermore, it was noted whether that descriptor was used as a criterion for subject inclusion in any particular group or if it was mentioned as additional subject information. Each type of descriptor was represented in at least one of the manuscripts. Rules for judging the presence or absence of a category were specified prior to reviewing the articles (see Appendix B). Generally, criteria for "presence" of a category were lenient. For example, if *any* physiological data were reported, that category would be judged as being present.

Reliability

In order to assess interjudge reliability, a second judge reviewed 15% of the manuscripts. Point-by-point reliability ranged from 82% to 100% when examined across descriptor variable groupings. Overall point-by-point agreement across all judgments was 96%.

RESULTS AND DISCUSSION

Subject Description

Subject description practices were examined by determining the degree to which researchers reported the 18 categories listed in Table 2. Figure 2 illustrates the percentage of manuscripts in which each descriptor was present. As might be predicted, more information regarding subjects is provided in the individual case studies, especially for some categories. The descriptors are listed in rank order of frequency of occurrence. Note that only three descriptors (medical diagnosis, age, and sex) occurred in more than 90% of the manuscripts.

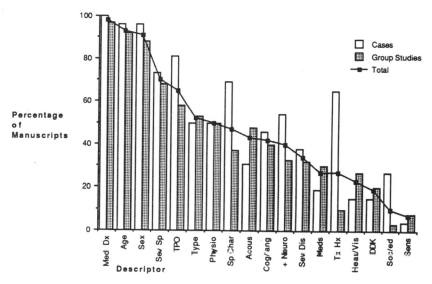

Figure 2. Percentage of manuscripts in which each descriptor was present. The group studies are indicated by the filled bars and the individual cases by the open bars. The total percentage for each descriptor is shown by the line graph.

Other potentially important information occurred less frequently. For example, indication of severity of the speech disorder (column "Sev Sp" in Figure 2) occurred in only 70% of the manuscripts reviewed. The criterion for presence of this descriptor was lenient and included even such general verbal descriptions as "most subjects were quite intelligible." Only 48% of the manuscripts indicated severity when a stricter criterion was used (e.g., 5- or 7-point rating scale or percent intelligibility measures). Time post-onset was noted in 65% of the manuscripts, but treatment history was noted in only 27% of the articles. When treatment history was noted, it was usually in individual case studies. Only six group studies (7%) reported whether the subjects had received or were receiving treatment.

Reported descriptors rarely included measures of diadochokinetic rate (19%), social or educational status (10%), and information regarding sensation (7%). Despite clinician report of usefulness (Gerratt, Till, Rosenbek, Wertz, & Boysen, 1991), DDK rates may not be seen as a useful descriptor of dysarthric speakers by those who contribute to clinical research literature. Likewise, social or educational status may not be pertinent in the majority of studies of individuals with dysarthria. It is much more difficult to understand the almost consistent failure to report sensory function. The fact that sensation is the least frequently reported of any descriptor may suggest that sensory and proprioceptive function are not considered important factors in the nature or treatment of dysarthria. Alternatively, it may be that investigators of clinical dysarthria simply do not have adequate measurement techniques to determine the integrity of the afferent systems.

. The presence or absence of any physiologic or acoustic data was also noted. Fewer than half (43%) of the articles reported acoustic data. It should be noted, however, that there was no consistency in the *type* of acoustic data reported. Because we noted only *presence* or *absence* of acoustic information, these results may indicate more consistency than actually exists. Acoustic data were reported primarily as dependent variables in the studies and rarely were used as subject descriptors or as criteria for group selection. Although almost 50% of manuscripts reported some physiologic information, there was little evidence for the use of a comprehensive physiologic protocol that compared performance across subsystems.

Subject Selection Criteria

One purpose of this chapter is to examine which subject variables were used as criteria for inclusion in a particular subject group. With a few exceptions, we found that particular criteria were never stated. Rather, subjects generally were grouped according to broad medical or speech classifications. In 61% of the articles reviewed, researchers used medical diagnosis as the classification for group comparisons (Figure 3). Examples of frequently reported subject groups were Parkinson's disease; amyotrophic lateral sclerosis (ALS); cerebral palsy, and traumatic brain injury.

The consistent dependence upon medical diagnosis for classification may be problematic for a number of reasons. First, speakers with the same medical diagnosis may form a heterogeneous group in terms of factors such as time post-onset and severity of dysarthria. Some medical diagnoses, such as traumatic brain injury, may result in a wide range of dysarthria types. Finally, speakers may vary greatly in patterns of respiratory, phonatory, and oral movement control, even within one medical diagnostic category.

Fewer than one quarter (22%) of the manuscripts grouped subjects according to type of dysarthria (Figure 3). Typically, these were hypokinetic or ataxic. In some of the articles, medical diagnosis and type of dysarthria were used as comparative subject groups in a particular study. For example, an ALS group might be compared with an ataxic dysarthric group on some dependent variable. This is very problematic, especially if the type of dysarthria exhibited by a particular ALS subject is not stated (e.g., primarily flaccid versus spastic). Some manuscripts (5%) grouped subjects only according to the label *dysarthric* versus *normal*, or *dysarthria* versus some other communicative disorder, such as conduction aphasia. Another 5% grouped subjects according to some feature of the dysarthria,

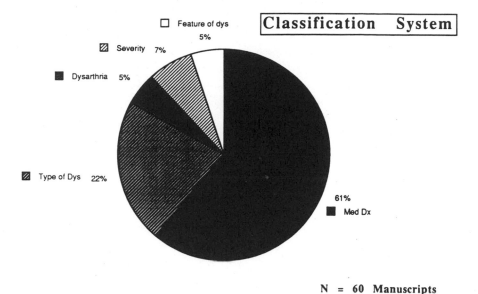

Figure 3. Classifications used for group comparisons. Percentages noted are those of total group studies in which that classification was used.

for example, "breathy voice." Only 7% of the articles used severity of the dysarthria to categorize groups or subjects.

Implications

This chapter focuses on several important questions relating to the progress of research in clinical dysarthria. Why are there so few published journal manuscripts in the area of clinical dysarthria? What are the consequences of lack of subject description in published articles? Why has there been such heavy reliance on medical diagnosis to classify subjects with dysarthria for group comparisons? How have practices of subject description and classification influenced interpretation of the data in dysarthria studies?

One striking finding of this review was the paucity of articles related to dysarthria. With the exception of editions of proceedings of biennial clinical dysarthria conferences, only 45 data-based articles appeared in the literature during the last 10 years. This is in stark contrast to the clinical research being reported for other communication disorders, such as stuttering. It is difficult, but important to account for this. It may be that university curricula emphasize the study of stuttering and other communication disorders, whereas less attention is given to dysarthria. Perhaps it is because the etiology of dysarthria is often quite explicit, whereas the cause for stuttering begs for investigation. Perhaps the relative dearth of published work in dysarthria is attributable to the general belief that treatment for dysarthria is only minimally effective. Distinct schools of treatment approaches for stuttering historically have competed in the research literature; however, treatment studies in dysarthria are few. More likely, the fact that so few manuscripts in clinical dysarthria exist is because research in the field has been clinically rather than theoretically driven. For example, the long history of theoretical controversy about *why* people stutter has led researchers to develop models and theories that prompt numerous investigations to provide data to support these positions. Researchers in clinical dysarthria have not yet developed such a broad theoretical framework. Until recently, the study of dysarthria has been primarily perceptually based and often descriptive. Advances in physiologic and acoustic measurements have provided increased opportunity to examine an increased variety of questions relating to motor speech disorders. Furthermore, the use of conceptual models of speech motor control as a basis for research in motor speech disorders may lead researchers to further investigations regarding the nature and treatment of dysarthria.

This chapter also illustrates the need to report more complete subject descriptions in order to facilitate interpretation of data. This is especially true in a field such as dysarthria where signs, symptoms, and severity differ widely. For example, is a group effect due to neurophysiologic differences in subject groups, or due to differences in severity? Subject description is also essential to the design and implementation of replication studies in dysarthria. Finally, lack of subject description greatly constrains the ability of the clinician to generalize interpretation of the data to his or her own patients. Information regarding specific subsystem involvement, levels of severity, and specific statements regarding speech and phonatory characteristics of the dysarthria allow the clinician to decide to what degree the data can be applied to patients who exhibit particular profiles of impairment. Subject description practices may be expected to vary depending upon the research question, yet such description should be in detail sufficient to allow replication of studies and to allow the clinical and research community to appreciate more fully speaker similarities and differences.

Comments regarding subject description apply primarily to investigations comparing group data. Subject description in individual case studies has usually been more specific and complete. This chapter indicates, however, that there exists little work that examines individual cases over time. Only a few studies have examined specific patterns of change in respiratory, phonatory, and articulatory performance in different speaking situations or contexts, or over time. Longitudinal studies examining the relative contribution of respiratory, laryngeal, and articulatory factors during periods of disease progression or during periods of spontaneous recovery and treatment have much to offer. Such work may offer insight regarding the efficacy of treatment and may aid in determining the physiologic and acoustic correlates of perceived intelligibility.

It has been said that one can learn a lot about persons' beliefs by observing their actions. This chapter suggests that what clinical researchers in dysarthria have done over the last 10 years is to rely most heavily on medical diagnosis to classify speakers with dysarthria. This may stem from the fact that clinicians who assess and treat patients with dysarthria have relied heavily on classification systems influenced primarily by the important work of Darley, Aronson, and Brown (1969a, 1969b, 1975). These classifications traditionally have focused on the perceptual characteristics of the speech motor control deficit associated with a particular disease or underlying pathophysiology. Our research indicates that because this frame of reference is so ingrained researchers tend to group subjects according to these medical classifications. What does this grouping of patients imply about beliefs held by researchers in this field? Such heavy reliance on medical diagnosis leads researchers to make a number of assumptions. First, it is assumed that the diagnosis is the most salient descriptor of dysarthric speakers. It is further assumed that one can make inferences about pathophysiology from the medical diagnosis. Finally, it is assumed that one can make inferences about approaches to intervention from the medical diagnosis. These three assumptions may well be accurate first order approximations of reality; however, one of the challenges of the next 10 years will be to question these assumptions.

The primary use of medical diagnosis as a classification system for dysarthric speakers has significant research implications. A fundamental issue in designing group research is the assignment of subjects to groups. This chapter suggests medical classifications have been carried over as the primary way to group subjects for comparison in between-group research designs in dysarthria. Depending upon the nature of the question, this may be appropriate (e.g., comparing the incidence of dysarthria in Parkinson's disease versus ALS). For many research questions, however, it makes more sense to group persons on factors other than medical diagnosis. For example, if the research question regards the laryngeal component of the dysarthria, it may be more appropriate to group patients on factors relating to respiratory and phonatory function versus etiology of the disorder. If one is interested in the impact of various augmentative communication approaches, it may make sense to group persons by severity of the speech impairment.

Future Directions

In conclusion, this chapter leads the researcher to consider several factors for continued research in clinical dysarthria. Specifically, we need to perform detailed perceptual physiologic and acoustic assessment within and across medical diagnosis in order to examine variability within and between populations. This will lead to research designs focused on examining groups of subjects who present with similar aerodynamic or movement performance deficits. We need more complete subject description to allow for replication studies and better interpretation of the data. We need in-depth analysis of individual subjects to examine the physiologic and acoustic parameters associated with perceptual deficits in intelligibility. Finally, we need to re-examine the use of medical diagnosis as the prevailing taxonomy in dysarthria research. Perhaps these steps will take us further toward the development and refinement of theories of speech motor control and motor speech disorders.

REFERENCES

Darley, F.L., Aronson, A.E., & Brown, J.R. (1969a). Differential diagnostic patterns of dysarthria. *Journal of Speech and Hearing Research, 12,* 246–269.

Darley, F.L., Aronson, A.E., & Brown, J.R. (1969b). Cluster of deviant speech dimensions in the dysarthrias. *Journal of Speech and Hearing Research, 12,* 462–496.

Darley, F.L., Aronson, A.E., & Brown, J.R. (1975). *Motor speech disorders.* Philadelphia: W.B. Saunders.

Gerratt, B.R., Till, J.A., Rosenbek, J.C., Wertz, R.T., & Boysen, A.E. (1991). Use and perceived value of perceptual and instrumental measures in dysarthria management. In C.A. Moore, K.M. Yorkston, & D.R. Beukelman (Eds.), *Dysarthria and apraxia of speech: Perspectives on management* (pp. 77–93). Baltimore: Paul H. Brookes Publishing Co.

Appendix A

Literature Sources

Journal of the Acoustical Society of America.

Forrest, K., Weismer, G., & Turner, G.S. (1989). Kinematic, acoustic, and perceptual analyses of connected speech produced by parkinsonian and normal geriatric adults. *Journal of the Acoustical Society of America*, 85, 2608–2622.

Gath, I., & Yair, E. (1988). Analysis of vocal tract parameters in parkinsonian speech. *Journal of the Acoustical Society of America*, 1628–1634.

Weismer, G., & Fennell, A.M. (1985). Constancy of (acoustic) relative timing measures in phrase-level utterances. *Journal of the Acoustical Society of America*, 78, 49–57.

Weismer, G., Kent, R.D., Hodge, M., & Martin, R. (1988). The acoustic signature for intelligibility test words. *Journal of the Acoustical Society of America*, 84, 1281–1291.

Brain and Language

Caliguiri, M.P. (1989). The influence of speaking rate on articulatory hypokinesia in parkinsonian dysarthria. *Brain and Language*, 36, 493–502.

Gentil, H. (1990). Dysarthria in Friedreich's disease. *Brain and Language*, 38, 438–448.

Kent, R.D., & Rosenbek, J.C. (1982). Prosodic disturbance and neurologic lesion. *Brain and Language*, 15, 259–291.

British Journal of Disorders of Communication

Enderby, P., & Crow, E. (1990). Long-term recovery patterns of severe dysarthria following head injury. *British Journal of Disorders of Communication*, 25, 341–354.

Hardcastle, W.J., Barry, R.A., & Clark, C.J. (1985). Articulatory and voicing characteristics of adult dysarthric and verbal dyspraxic speakers: An instrumental study. *British Journal of Disorders of Communication*, 20, 249–270.

Johnson, J.A., & Pring, T.R. (1990). Speech therapy and Parkinson's disease: A review and further data. *British Journal of Disorders of Communication*, 25, 183–194.

Kallen, D., Marshall, R.C., & Casey, D.E. (1986). Atypical dysarthria in Munchausen syndrome. *British Journal of Disorders of Communication*, 21, 377–380.

Pitcairn, T.K., Clemie, S., Gray, J.M., & Pentlund, B. (1990). Impressions of parkinsonian patients from their recorded voices. *British Journal of Disorders of Communication*, 25, 85–92.

Robertson, S.J., & Thomson, F. (1984). Speech therapy in Parkinson's disease: A study of the efficacy and long-term effects of intensive treatment. *British Journal of Disorders of Communication*, 19, 213–224.

Ziegler, W., & Von Cramon, D. (1986). Spastic dysarthria after acquired brain injury: An acoustic study. *British Journal of Disorders of Communication, 21,* 173–187.

Clinical Dysarthria

Ansel, B.M., McNeil, M.R., Hunker, C.J., & Bless, D.M. (1983). The frequency of verbal and acoustic adjustments used by cerebral palsied dysarthric adults when faced with communicative failure. In W. Berry (Ed.), *Clinical dysarthria.* Boston: College-Hill.

Berry, W., & Goshorn, E. (1983). Immediate visual feedback in the treatment of ataxic dysarthria: A case study. In W. Berry (Ed.), *Clinical dysarthria.* Boston: College-Hill.

Caliguiri, M.P., & Murry, T. (1983). The use of visual feedback to enhance prosodic control in dysarthria. In W. Berry (Ed.), *Clinical dysarthria.* Boston: College-Hill.

DeFeo, A.B., & Schaefer, C.M. (1983). Bilateral facial paralysis in a preschool child: Oral-facial and articulatory characteristics (A case study). In W. Berry (Ed.), *Clinical dysarthria.* Boston: College-Hill.

Hanson, W., & Metter, E. (1983). DAF speech rate modification in Parkinson's disease: A report of two cases. In W. Berry (Ed.), *Clinical dysarthria.* Boston: College-Hill.

Ludlow, C.L., & Bassich, C.J. (1983). The results of acoustic and perceptual assessment of two types of dysarthria. In W. Berry (Ed.), *Clinical dysarthria.* Boston: College-Hill.

McNamara, R.D. (1983). A conceptual holistic approach to dysarthria treatment. In W. Berry (Ed.), *Clinical dysarthria.* Boston: College-Hill.

Murry, T. (1983). The production of stress in three types of dysarthric speech. In W. Berry (Ed.), *Clinical dysarthria.* Boston: College-Hill.

Shaugnessy, A., Netsell, R., & Farrage, J. (1983). Treatment of a four year old with a palatal lift prosthesis. In W. Berry (Ed.), *Clinical dysarthria.* Boston: College-Hill.

Simmons, N. (1983). Acoustic analysis of ataxic dysarthria: An approach to monitoring treatment. In W. Berry (Ed.), *Clinical dysarthria.* Boston: College-Hill.

Yorkston, K.M., & Beukelman, D.R. (1983). The influence of judge familiarization with the speaker on dysarthric speech intelligibility. In W. Berry (Ed.), *Clinical dysarthria.* Boston: College-Hill.

Dysarthria and Apraxia of Speech: Perspectives on Management

Barkmeier, J., Jordon, L.S., Robin, D.A., & Schum, R.L. (1991). Inexperienced listener ratings of dysarthric speaker intelligibility and physical appearance. In C.A. Moore, K.M. Yorkston, & D.R. Beukelman (Eds.), *Dysarthria and apraxia of speech: Perspectives on management.* Baltimore: Paul H. Brookes Publishing Co.

Forrest, K., Adams, S., McNeil, M.R., & Southwood, H. (1991). Kinematic, electromyographic, and perceptual evaluation of speech apraxia, conduction aphasia, ataxic dysarthria, and normal speech production. In C.A. Moore, K.M. Yorkston, & D.R. Beukelman (Eds.), *Dysarthria and apraxia of speech: Perspectives on management.* Baltimore: Paul H. Brookes Publishing Co.

Hammen, V.L., Yorkston, K.M., & Dowden, P. (1991). Index of contextual intelligibility I: Impact of semantic context in dysarthria. In C.A. Moore, K.M. Yorkston, & D.R. Beukelman (Eds.), *Dysarthria and apraxia of speech: Perspectives on management.* Baltimore: Paul H. Brookes Publishing Co.

Metter, E.J., & Hanson, W.R. (1991). Dysarthria in progressive supranuclear palsy. In C.A. Moore, K.M. Yorkston, & D.R. Beukelman (Eds.), *Dysarthria and apraxia of speech: Perspectives on management.* Baltimore: Paul H. Brookes Publishing Co.

Robin, D.A., & Eliason, M.J. (1991). Speech and prosodic problems in children with neurofibromatosis. In C.A. Moore, K.M. Yorkston, & D.R. Beukelman (Eds.), *Dysarthria and apraxia of speech: Perspectives on management.* Baltimore: Paul H. Brookes Publishing Co.

Robin, D.A., Somodi, L.B., & Luschei, E.S. (1991). Measurement of tongue strength and endurance in normal and articulation disordered subjects. In C.A. Moore, K.M. Yorkston, & D.R. Beukelman (Eds.), *Dysarthria and apraxia of speech: Perspectives on management.* Baltimore: Paul H. Brookes Publishing Co.

Schulz, G.M., & Ludlow, C.L. (1991). Botulinum treatment for orolingual-mandibular dystonia: Speech effects. In C.A. Moore, K.M. Yorkston, & D.R. Beukelman (Eds.), *Dysarthria and apraxia of speech: Perspectives on management.* Baltimore: Paul H. Brookes Publishing Co.

Stuart, S.L., Beukelman, D.R., Kenyon, K.K., Healey, E.C., & Bernthal, J.E. (1991). Dysarthria following Reye's syndrome: A case report. In C.A. Moore, K.M. Yorkston, & D.R. Beukelman (Eds.), *Dysarthria and apraxia of speech: Perspectives on management.* Baltimore: Paul H. Brookes Publishing Co.

Till, J.A., & Alp, L.A. (1991). Aerodynamic and temporal measures of continuous speech in dysarthric speakers. In C.A. Moore, K.M. Yorkston, & D.R. Beukelman (Eds.), *Dysarthria and apraxia of speech: Perspectives on management.* Baltimore: Paul H. Brookes Publishing Co.

Workinger, M.S., & Kent, R.D. (1991). Perceptual analysis of the dysarthrias in children with athetoid and spastic cerebral palsy. In C.A. Moore, K.M. Yorkston, & D.R. Beukelman (Eds.), *Dysarthria and apraxia of speech: Perspectives on management.* Baltimore: Paul H. Brookes Publishing Co.

Yorkston, K.M., Hammen, V.L., & Dowden, P.A. (1991). Index of contextual intelligibility: A perceptual analysis of intelligible versus unintelligible productions in severe dysarthria. In C.A. Moore, K.M. Yorkston, & D.R. Beukelman (Eds.), *Dysarthria and apraxia of speech: Perspectives on management.* Baltimore: Paul H. Brookes Publishing Co.

Dysarthrias: Physiology, Acoustics, Perception, Management

Aten, J., McDonald, A., Simpson, M., & Gutierrez, R. (1984). Efficacy of modified palatal lifts for improved resonance. In M. McNeil, J. Rosenbek, & A. Aronson (Eds.), *Dysarthrias: Physiology, acoustics, perception, management.* Austin, TX: PRO-ED.

Hunker, C.J., & Abbs, J.H. (1984). Physiological analyses of parkinsonian tremors in the orofacial system. In M. McNeil, J. Rosenbek, & A. Aronson (Eds.), *Dysarthrias: Physiology, acoustics, perception, management.* Austin, TX: PRO-ED.

Linebaugh, C.W., & Wolfe, V.E. (1984). Relationships between articulation rate, intelligibility, and naturalness in spastic and ataxic speakers. In M. McNeil, J. Rosenbek, & A. Aronson (Eds.), *Dysarthrias: Physiology, acoustics, perception, management.* Austin, TX: PRO-ED.

Ludlow, C., & Bassich, C. (1984). Relationships between perceptual ratings and acoustic measures of hypokinetic speech. In M. McNeil, J. Rosenbek, & A. Aronson (Eds.), *Dysarthrias: Physiology, acoustics, perception, management.* Austin, TX: PRO-ED.

Rubow, R. (1984). Role of feedback, reinforcement, and compliance on training and transfer in biofeedback-based rehabilitation of motor speech disorders. In M. McNeil, J. Rosenbek, & A. Aronson (Eds.), *Dysarthrias: Physiology, acoustics, perception, management.* Austin, TX: PRO-ED.

Weismer, G. (1984). Articulatory characteristics of parkinsonian dysarthria: Segmental and phrase-level timing, spirantization, and glottal-supraglottal coordination. In M. McNeil, J. Rosenbek, & A. Aronson (Eds.), *Dysarthrias: Physiology, acoustics, perception, management.* Austin, TX: PRO-ED.

Yorkston, K.M., Beukelman, D.R., Minifie, F., & Sapir, S. (1984). Assessment of stress patterning. In M. McNeil, J. Rosenbek, & A. Aronson (Eds.), *Dysarthrias: Physiology, acoustics, perception, management.* Austin, TX: PRO-ED.

Folia Phoniatrica

Hirose, H., Kiritani, S., & Sawashima, M. (1982). Patterns of dysarthric movement in patients with amyotrophic lateral sclerosis and pseudobulbar palsy. *Folia Phoniatrica, 34,* 106–112.

Hirose, H., Kiritani, S., & Sawashima, M. (1982). Velocity of articulatory movements in normal and dysarthric subjects. *Folia Phoniatrica, 34,* 210–215.

Schliesser, H. (1982). Alternate motion rates of the speech articulators in adults with cerebral palsy. *Folia Phoniatrica, 34,* 258–264.

Journal of Communication Disorders

Bedwinek, A.P., & O'Brian, R.L. (1985). A patient selection profile for the use of speech prosthesis in adult disorders. *Journal of Communication Disorders, 18,* 169–182.

Bellaire, K., Yorkston, K.M., & Beukelman, D.R. (1986). Modification of breath patterning to increase naturalness of a mildly dysarthric speaker. *Journal of Communication Disorders, 19,* 271–280.

Canter, G.J., & Van Lanker, D. (1985). Disturbance of the temporal organization of speech following bilateral thalamic surgery in a patient with Parkinson's disease. *Journal of Communication Disorders, 18,* 371–391.

Day, L.S., & Parnell, M.M. (1987). Ten year study of a Wilson's disease dysarthric. *Journal of Communication Disorders, 20,* 207–218.

Dworkin, J., & Aronson, A. (1986). Tongue strength and alternate motion rates in normal and dysarthric subjects. *Journal of Communication Disorders, 19,* 115–132.

Hoodin, R.B., & Gilbert, H.R. (1989). Nasal airflows in parkinsonian speakers. *Journal of Communication Disorders, 22,* 169–180.

LaBlance, G.R., & Rutherford, D.R. (1991). Respiratory dynamics and speech intelligibility in speakers with generalized dystonia. *Journal of Communication Disorders, 24,* 141–156.

Metter, E.J., & Hanson, W.R. (1986). Clinical and acoustical variability in hypokinetic dysarthria. *Journal of Communication Disorders, 19,* 347–366.

Morris, R. (1989). Voice onset time and dysarthria: A descriptive study. *Journal of Communication Disorders, 22,* 23–33.

Seikel, J.A., Wilcox, K.A., & Davis, J. (1990). Dysarthria of motor neuron disease: Clinician judgements of severity. *Journal of Communication Disorders, 23,* 417–431.

Journal of Speech and Hearing Disorders

Barlow, A., & Abbs, J. (1983). Force transducers for the evaluation of labial, lingual, and mandibular motor impairments. *Journal of Speech and Hearing Disorders, 26,* 616.

Kent, R.D., Kent, J.F., Weismer, G., Sufit, R.L., Rosenbek, J.C., Martin, R.E., & Brooks, B.R. (1990). Impairment of speech intelligibility in men with amyotrophic lateral sclerosis. *Journal of Speech and Hearing Disorders, 55,* 721–728.

Kent, R.D., Weismer, G., Kent, J.F., & Rosenbek, J.C. (1989). Toward phonetic intelligibility testing in dysarthria. *Journal of Speech and Hearing Disorders, 54,* 482–499.

Murdoch, B.E., Chenery, H.J., Bowler, S., & Ingram, J.C.L. (1989). Respiratory function in Parkinson's subjects exhibiting a perceptible speech deficit: A kinematic and spirometric analysis. *Journal of Speech and Hearing Disorders, 54,* 610–626.

Portnoy, R.A., & Aronson, A.E. (1982). Diadochokinetic syllable rate and regularity in normal and in spastic ataxic dysarthric subjects. *Journal of Speech and Hearing Disorders, 47,* 324–328.

Ramig, L.O., Scherer, R.C., Klasner, E.R., Titze, I.R., & Horii, Y. (1990). Acoustic analysis of voice in amyotrophic lateral sclerosis: A longitudinal case study. *Journal of Speech and Hearing Disorders, 55,* 2–14.

Simpson, M.B., Till, J.A., & Goff, A.M. (1988). Long-term treatment of severe dysarthria: A case study. *Journal of Speech and Hearing Disorders, 53,* 433–440.

Till, J.A., & Toye, A.R. (1988). Acoustic phonetic effects of two types of verbal feedback in dysarthric subjects. *Journal of Speech and Hearing Disorders, 53,* 449–458.

Yorkston, K.M., Hammen, V.L., Beukelman, D.R., & Traynor, C.D. (1990). The effect of rate control on the intelligibility and naturalness of dysarthric speech. *Journal of Speech and Hearing Disorders, 55,* 550–561.

Journal of Speech and Hearing Research

Barlow, S.M., & Burton, M.S. (1990). Ramp-and-hold force control in the upper and lower lips: Developing new neuromotor assessment applications in traumatic brain injured adults. *Journal of Speech and Hearing Research, 33,* 660–675.

Barlow, S.M., Cole, K., & Abbs, J. (1983). A new head-mounted lip-jaw movement transduction system for the study of motor speech disorders. *Journal of Speech and Hearing Research, 26,* 283–288.

McClean, M.D., Beukelman, D.R., & Yorkston, K.M. (1987). Speech-muscle visuomotor tracking in dysarthric and nonimpaired speakers. *Journal of Speech and Hearing Research, 30,* 276–282.

McNeil, M.R., Weismer, G., Adams, S., & Mulligan, M. (1990). Oral structure nonspeech motor control in normal, dysarthric, aphasic and apraxic speakers: Postural force and position. *Journal of Speech and Hearing Research, 33,* 255–268.

Murdoch, B.E., Chenery, H.J., Stokes, P.D., & Hardcastle, W.H. (1991). Respiratory kinematics in speakers with cerebellar disease. *Journal of Speech and Hearing Research, 34,* 768–780.

Neilson, P., & O'Dwyer, N. (1984). Reproducibility and variability of speech muscle activity in athetoid dysarthria of cerebral palsy. *Journal of Speech and Hearing Research, 27,* 502–517.

Odell, K., McNeil, M.R., Rosenbek, J.C., & Hunter, L. (1991). Perceptual characteristics of vowel and prosody productions in apraxic, aphasic, and dysarthric speakers. *Journal of Speech and Hearing Research, 34,* 60–66.

O'Dwyer, N., Neilson, P., Guitar, B.E., Quinn, P.T., & Andrews, G. (1983). Control of upper airway structures during nonspeech tasks in normal and cerebral-palsied subjects: EMG findings. *Journal of Speech and Hearing Research, 26,* 162–170.

Sheard, C., Adams, R.D., & Davis, P.J. (1991). Reliability and agreement of ratings of ataxic dysarthric speech samples with varying intelligibility. *Journal of Speech and Hearing Research, 34,* 285–293.

Recent Advances in Clinical Dysarthria

Barlow, S.M., & Netsell, R. (1989). Clinical neurophysiology for individuals with dysarthria. In K.M. Yorkston & D.R. Beukelman (Eds.), *Recent advances in clinical dysarthria.* Austin, TX: PRO-ED.

Caligiuri, M.P. (1989). Short-term fluctuations in orofacial motor control in Parkinson's disease. In K.M. Yorkston & D.R. Beukelman (Eds.), *Recent advances in clinical dysarthria.* Austin, TX: PRO-ED.

Crow, E., & Enderby, P. (1989). The effects of an alphabet chart on the speaking rate and intelligibility of speakers with dysarthria. In K.M. Yorkston & D.R. Beukelman (Eds.), *Recent advances in clinical dysarthria.* Austin, TX: PRO-ED.

Daniel-Whitney, B. (1989). Severe spastic-ataxic dysarthria in a child with traumatic brain injury: Questions for management. In K.M. Yorkston & D.R. Beukelman (Eds.), *Recent advances in clinical dysarthria.* Austin, TX: PRO-ED.

Hammen, V.L., Yorkston, K.M., & Beukelman, D.R. (1989). Pausal and speech duration characteristics as a function of speaking rate in normal and dysarthric individuals. In K.M. Yorkston & D.R. Beukelman (Eds.), *Recent advances in clinical dysarthria.* Austin, TX: PRO-ED.

Hartman, D.E., & O'Neill, B.P. (1989). Progressive dysfluency, dysphagia, dysarthria: A case of olivopontocerebellar atrophy. In K.M. Yorkston & D.R. Beukelman (Eds.), *Recent advances in clinical dysarthria.* Austin, TX: PRO-ED.

Lotz, W., & Netsell, R. (1989). Velopharyngeal management for a child with dysarthria and cerebral palsy. In K.M. Yorkston & D.R. Beukelman (Eds.), *Recent advances in clinical dysarthria.* Austin, TX: PRO-ED.

Moore, C.A., & Scudder, R.R. (1989). Coordination of jaw muscle activity in parkinsonian movement: Description and response to traditional treatment. In K.M. Yorkston & D.R. Beukelman (Eds.), *Recent advances in clinical dysarthria.* Austin, TX: PRO-ED.

Philippbar, S.A., Robin, D.A., & Luschei, E.S. (1989). Limb, jaw, and vocal tremor in Parkinson's patients. In K.M. Yorkston & D.R. Beukelman (Eds.), *Recent advances in clinical dysarthria.* Austin, TX: PRO-ED.

Vogel, D. (1989). Effects of thyrotropin-releasing hormone on dysarthria in amyotrophic lateral sclerosis. In K.M. Yorkston & D.R. Beukelman (Eds.), *Recent advances in clinical dysarthria.* Austin, TX: PRO-ED.

Yorkston, K.M., Honsinger, M.J., Beukelman, D.R., & Taylor, T. (1989). The effects of palatal lift fitting on the perceived articulatory adequacy of dysarthric speakers. In K.M. Yorkston & D.R. Beukelman (Eds.), *Recent advances in clinical dysarthria.* Austin, TX: PRO-ED.

Appendix B

Rules for Judging Presence or Absence of the Descriptor

Acoustic data:	Any data involving acoustic analysis of speech
Age:	Age of subject or subjects was provided. For the group studies, it was sufficient to provide the mean age with an indication of the range.
Cognition and language:	Any test scores or general description of subject's intellectual status or language skills
Diadochokinesis:	Either verbal description of rapid alternating movement rates or objective measures of diadochokinesis (DDK) rates
Disease severity:	Any indication of severity of etiologic disorder (e.g., staging of Parkinson's disease with Hoehn and Yahr scale)
Hearing and vision:	Any mention of *either* hearing or vision acuity or perception
Medical diagnosis:	Any indication of underlying etiology
Medications:	Any indication of current medications
Neurologic exam data:	Neurologic description or information in addition to diagnosis (e.g., CT scan)
Physiologic data:	Any data related to physiology of respiratory, laryngeal, velopharyngeal, or articulatory processes
Sensation:	Any indication of a sensory exam being completed
Severity of dysarthria:	Very lenient with this to get a conservative description For example we saw many statements such as "most subjects were quite intelligible" or "subjects represented a broad range of severity." These were counted as providing severity information although very little information regarding severity was conveyed.
Sex:	Gender of subjects
Socioeconomic status and education:	Any indication of occupation, social status, or years of education
Speech characteristics:	Any verbal description of speech characteristics (e.g., harsh voice; imprecise consonant production)

Time post-onset: Any indication of duration of the speech or medical problem

Treatment history: Any description of course of intervention

Type of dysarthria: Any indication of perceptually derived types of dysarthria (e.g., ataxic or mixed flaccid/spastic)

SECTION II

CLINICAL CHARACTERISTICS

Chapter 4

Perceptual–Acoustic Speech and Voice Characteristics of Subjects with Spasmodic Torticollis

Leonard L. LaPointe,
James L. Case, and Drake D. Duane

DYSTONIA IS A neurogenic disorder of posture and movement characterized by abnormal muscle contractions frequently accompanied by regular or irregular twisting or repetitive movements. These abnormal postures and movements can be sustained or intermittent and can be present in many parts of the body or in selected focal body parts when either at rest or during voluntary motor activity (Scientific Advisory Board of the Dystonia Medical Research Foundation, 1988). Approximately three fourths of patients diagnosed with dystonia have an idiopathic primary dystonia that can be inherited or sporadic, the remainder have symptomatic or secondary dystonias associated with a variety of neuropathologies, including trauma and iatrogenic drug-induced etiologies (Fahn, Marsden, & Calne, 1988). Classification of dystonia relative to body distribution includes generalized dystonia, affecting one or both legs plus another area of the body; segmental dystonia, affecting two or more contiguous areas of the body; and focal dystonia, where only one area or part of the body is affected.

Focal dystonias include abnormal contraction and movement of the muscles of the eye (blepharospasm), the mouth and face (oromandibular), the hand ("writer's cramp"), the larynx (adductor and abductor spasmodic dysphonia), and the strap muscles of the neck (spasmodic torticollis).

SPASMODIC TORTICOLLIS

An ongoing, larger study of the acoustic, speech, and other behavioral characteristics of dystonias has enabled our research to focus on a large subsample of subjects with spasmodic torticollis. This focal dystonia is characterized by hypercontractions of the neck muscles that typically cause an involuntary posture or deviation of the head from normal position. This also has been referred to as cervical dystonia. Spasmodic torticollis is the most common form of focal dystonia (McGeer & McGeer, 1988). Few studies exist of large samples of the clinical features of subjects with spasmodic torticollis, although Duane (1988) compiled epidemiological data on 347 patients seen at the Mayo Clinic. He reported that female patients outnumbered males at 1.6 to 1.0; the mean age at onset was approximately 43 years; a positive family history of dystonia or essential tremor existed in 10% of the sample; non–right-handedness was rare; and light eyes (blue, green, or hazel) were characteristics of the preponderance of subjects.

Speech and Voice Characteristics

Because the affected muscles in spasmodic torticollis surround the critical region of the larynx, and because it has been observed clinically that aberrations of movement and posture of the neck can flow over into other functional components of the speech production mechanism, it is surprising that so few studies of the effects of spasmodic characteristics on speech and voice exist. A few clinical observations of vocal involvement can be found scattered throughout the literature on dystonia. For example, Blitzer and Brin (1991) commented on "vocal involvement" of focal dystonic subjects; Kammermeier (1969) reported vocal frequency, intensity, and durational measures obtained from speech samples of eight dystonic subjects; and Darley, Aronson, and Brown (1975) reported some perceptual speech and voice characteristics of 30 subjects with dystonia. Two studies of orolingual-mandibular dystonia (Golper, Nutt, Rau, & Coleman, 1983; Schulz & Ludlow, 1991) also reported on the characteristics of a focal dystonia. Additionally Schulz and Ludlow reported the results of treating this focal dystonia with localized injections of *Botulinum A toxin* (Botox). To date, we have found no detailed report of acoustic-perceptual analyses of the speech and voice characteristics of subjects with spasmodic torticollis. In a continuing collaborative project between the Arizona Dystonia Institute and Arizona State University, we have now evaluated over 250 subjects with dystonia. This chapter presents the results of our research on a subsample of 70 subjects with spasmodic torticollis. Some of the acoustic voice characteristics of this sample have been reported previously (Case, LaPointe, & Duane, 1990; Duane, Case, & LaPointe, 1991; LaPointe, Case, & Duane, 1990).

Methods

Seventy subjects (25 males, 45 females) were included in the subsample of individuals with dystonia in this study. The subjects were selected because all fulfilled the diagnostic criteria of spasmodic torticollis and analysis of their speech-voice characteristics had been completed. All subjects were diagnosed with spasmodic torticollis by the third author, a neurologist at the Arizona Dystonia Institute. Severity and specific characteristics of the focal dystonia were judged and an array of behavioral and neurologic evaluative measures were included in the basic evaluation protocol of each subject. Mean age of the subjects was 52.2 years. Twenty subjects (7 males, 13 females) who self-reported to be free of neurological disease or history were matched for gender and age and served as a control group for comparison across an array of dependent speech and acoustic variables.

A standardized protocol designed to elicit a range of movement, speech, vocal, and communication behaviors was used with each subject, and responses to this protocol were both audio- and videotape recorded. Audio recordings were made with a Marantz 430 recorder and all voice and speech samples were obtained using a microphone-to-subject distance of 10 cm. Only the audio recordings were analyzed for this study. Analysis was done using a microcomputer-based analog-to-digital converter (MicroSpeech Lab) with a digitizing rate of 10,000 Hertz. This sampling rate was greater than two and one half times the highest fundamental frequency (Fo) obtained from the sample, and was judged to be adequate for the study. For determining reliability, approximately five percent of the tested variables were re-analyzed at a later date (from 2 to 10 weeks) using the Kay Elemetrics Digital 5500 Sonograph using a 20,000 Hertz sampling rate. If the sample obtained was within 5 Hz (plus or minus), agreement was accepted. Accuracy of the re-analyzed sample for reliability of original measurements was 100%, using these criteria.

Eighteen parameters of these speech and voice behaviors were selected for analysis and served as the comparative dependent variables between the group with spasmodic torticollis and the control groups.

1. Reading rate (words per minute)
2. Duration of /s/ sound (seconds)
3. Duration of /z/ sound (seconds)
4. /s/, /z/ duration ratio
5. Maximum phonation duration (MPD) of vowel /a/ (seconds)
6. Habitual speaking frequency (HSFo) during counting from 5 to 10 (Hz)

7. Basal sustained fundamental frequency (BFo)
8. Ceiling sustained fundamental frequency (CFo)
9. Fundamental frequency range (Hz)
10. Sequential movement rate (SMR) for lips (/p∧/), syllables per second
11. SMR for tongue tip (/t∧/), syllables per second
12. SMR for tongue back (/k∧/), syllables per second
13. Alternate movement rate (AMR) for lips, tongue tip, tongue back (/p∧t∧k∧/), syllables per second
14. Contrastive stress accuracy index [CSAI], (/p∧/)
15. Contrastive stress accuracy index [CSAI], (/t∧/)
16. Contrastive stress accuracy index [CSAI], (/k∧/)
17. Phonation reaction time (PRT)
18. Intelligibility rating (7-point equal appearing interval scale)

Instructions for the elicitation of all speech and voice parameters were standardized across subjects, with modeling of each speech or voice parameter by the examiner. Whenever maximal performance was required several trials were used (three, for most attempts) and the optimal of the multiple attempts was used. Because instructions can have a strong effect on performance (Kent, Kent, & Rosenbek, 1987), every attempt was made to maintain uniform instructions across subjects.

Measurements and coding of the data for each subject were preserved on specially designed subject data sheets and then subjected to a variety of descriptive and inferential statistical analyses.

RESULTS AND DISCUSSION

Statistically significant differences (Unpaired t-test, $p < .05$) were found between the performances of subjects with spasmodic torticollis and control subjects across several of the speech and voice parameters measured. Although total alpha level may be influenced by running a large number of t-tests, we were comfortable with the results of our analysis, given the very large differences obtained. These differences are summarized in Table 1.

Differences Across Variables

As can be seen in Table 1, significant differences were found for 13 of the 18 speech and voice variables between spasmodic torticollis and control subjects. Subjects with spasmodic torticollis tended to have slower speech and movement rates as manifested on many of the tasks. As a group, the spasmodic torticollis subjects read approximately 30 words per minute slower than the control subjects. Duration data also indicated shorter values for /s/, /z/, and /a/ prolongation for the subjects with spasmodic

Table 1. Performance means, standard deviations, and levels of significant difference between spasmodic torticollis and control subjects

Variable	ST subjects		Control subjects		Significance
	Mean	SD	Mean	SD	
Reading rate (wpm)	164.7	33.4	194.6	17.9	0.0003*
/s/ duration (sec)	15.3	7.2	22.3	7.4	0.0001*
/z/ duration (sec)	18.7	8.0	25.8	7.1	0.0003*
MPD of /a/ (sec)	16.57	7.1	20.9	4.6	0.01*
SMR lips (sec)	5.08	1.1	6.6	0.9	0.0001*
SMR tongue tip (sec)	4.83	1.2	6.4	1.0	0.0001*
SMR tongue back (sec)	4.47	1.1	6.0	0.8	0.0001*
AMR /p$\wedge$t$\wedge$K$\wedge$/ (sec)	4.79	1.3	6.9	0.9	0.0001*
Intelligibility rating	5.68	2.2	7.0	0.0	0.016*
HSFo females (Hz)	169.7	41.6	190.6	40.4	0.02*
CFo females (Hz)	551.2	235.7	964.5	281.0	0.0001*
Fo range females (Hz)	407.5	222.4	809.8	260.0	0.0001*
PRT males and females (ms)	544.0	165.0	355	97.0	0.0001*

torticollis. The alternate and sequential movement rates generated by repetition of /p$\wedge$/, /t$\wedge$/, /k$\wedge$/, and /p$\wedge$ t$\wedge$ k$\wedge$/ revealed subjects' abilities to sequence rapidly the motor speech components of respiration, phonation, and various articulatory components of the upper airway. Subjects with spasmodic torticollis had somewhat more difficulty and performed more slowly than control subjects.

Phonatory Comparisons

The phonatory parameters revealed several interesting findings when performances were compared. It is well known that male and female subjects can be expected to perform differently on vocal parameters, especially regarding pitch; therefore, subject performances were not pooled across gender for these analyses. Females with spasmodic torticollis tended to have lower fundamental frequencies of habitual speaking levels, as well as lower ceiling fundamental frequencies, than female speakers in the control group. Overall, the phonatory pitch performance of the subjects with spasmodic torticollis seemed to be shifted downward along all parameters. This was confirmed by the fundamental frequency shifts in ceiling, as well as habitual speaking levels. For example, the group mean habitual speaking fundamental frequency for the female subjects with spasmodic torticollis was 169.7 Hz compared to 190.6 Hz for the control female subjects.

Perhaps the most remarkable phonatory difference between subject groups was on the ceiling fundamental frequency data for females. Female subjects with spasmodic torticollis as a group produced a mean ceiling fundamental frequency of 551.2 Hz, compared to 964.6 Hz for the control female subjects. This difference seems to indicate that spasmodic torticollis in female subjects reduces maximal fundamental frequency capabilities by nearly one full octave.

Phonatory Reaction Time

A final phonatory difference that emerged between groups was on phonatory reaction time. There was no reason to believe that males and females would perform differently for this task, so performance across gender was pooled. A sound field "click" was produced approximately 20 cm from each subject. Subjects were instructed to keep their eyes closed for this task and to produce an /a/ sound as quickly as possible after hearing the "click" signal. Three trials were given and the shortest latency in milliseconds was selected between the "click" and phonatory onset. Subjects with spasmodic torticollis produced a mean PRT of 544 ms, significantly slower than the mean of 355 ms produced by the control subjects.

Although both the subjects with spasmodic torticollis and the control subjects had speech that was perceived to be intelligible, slight differences occurred in the mean ratings on the 7-point equal appearing interval scale between groups. All control subjects were judged to have the highest perceived rating of intelligibility; that is, a score of 7.00, whereas subjects with spasmodic torticollis were judged to have a group mean intelligibility rating of 5.68. No subject with spasmodic torticollis was judged to have unintelligible speech, and the overall clinical impression of the speech of those with spasmodic torticollis was that it was functional and intelligible, even if subtly different along some parameters.

SUMMARY AND CONCLUSIONS

This chapter provides the first detailed analysis and report of perceptual and acoustic speech variables associated with cervical dystonia or spasmodic torticollis. Although the overall clinical impression of the speech and voice of many of these subjects might lead an examiner to the inference that either subclinical or no significant impairment is associated with this focal dystonia, careful acoustic and perceptual analysis has revealed several differences. These differences are especially apparent along the variables related to fundamental frequency, sequential and alternate movement rates, sibilant and vowel duration, and phonation reaction time. The torque-like deviations of posture that affect the muscles and structures that house the laryngeal and upper airway components of the speech production system, indeed, influence speech and voice parameters.

We have had the good fortune to form a productive collaborative clinical research relationship between the speech physiology and voice laboratory of Arizona State University and the Arizona Dystonia Institute. Currently we have collected data on over 250 subjects with a variety of focal and segmental dystonias. Our continuing investigations will attempt to define further speech-voice relationships with neurologic and behavioral factors. We have completed study of postural-mechanical influences on speech and voice parameters of nondisabled control subjects, as well as on perturbation measures of subjects with dystonia. The effects of specific treatment paradigms, such as focal injection of *Botulinum A toxin* (Botox), are also under investigation. These descriptions, observed differences, and continuing investigations will begin to map the territory of the influence of these disorders on speech motor control and may serve to refine understanding of the nature and course of these puzzling aberrations of movement and posture. More importantly, perhaps, advances in understanding these movement disorders will aid those involved in clinical management of persons with spasmodic torticollis.

REFERENCES

Blitzer, A., & Brin, F. (1991). Laryngeal dystonia: A series with botulinum toxin therapy. *Annals of Otology, Rhinology and Laryngology, 100*, 85–89.

Case, J., LaPointe, L., & Duane, D. (1990). Speech and voice characteristics in spasmodic torticollis. Paper presented at the International Congress of Movement Disorders, Washington, DC. (Abstract in *Movement Disorders, 5*, 1990, 84).

Darley, F., Aronson, A., & Brown, J. (1975). *Motor speech disorders.* Philadelphia: W.B. Saunders.

Duane, D. (1988). Spasmodic torticollis: Clinical and biological features and the implications for focal dystonia. In S. Fahn, C. Marsden, & D. Calne (Eds.), *Advances in neurology: Vol. 50. Dystonia 2.* New York: Raven Press.

Duane, D., Case, J., & LaPointe, L. (1991) Patterns of dystonia, tremor, voice, and lateralization in cervical dystonia. Paper presented at the American Academy of Neurology, Miami. (Abstract in *Annals of Neurology, 30*, 259).

Fahn S., Marsden, C., & Calne, D. (Eds.). (1988) *Advances in neurology: 50. Dystonia 2.* New York: Raven Press.

Golper, L., Nutt, J., Rau, M., & Coleman, R. (1983). Focal cranial dystonia. *Journal of Speech and Hearing Disorders, 48*, 128–134.

Kammermeier, M.A. (1969). *A comparison of phonatory phenomena among groups of neurologically impaired speakers.* Unpublished doctoral dissertation, University of Minnesota.

Kent, R.D., Kent, J.F., & Rosenbek, J.C. (1987). Maximum performance tests of speech production. *Journal of Speech and Hearing Disorders, 52*, 367–387.

LaPointe, L.L., Case, J.L., & Duane, D. (1990). *Perceptual and acoustic vocal characteristics of subjects with spasmodic torticollis.* Paper presented at the annual convention of American Speech-Language-Hearing Association, Seattle.

McGeer, E., & McGeer, P. (1988). The dystonias. *Canadian Journal of Neurological Sciences, 15*, 447–483.

Schulz, G.M., & Ludlow, C.L. (1991). Botulinum treatment for orolingual-mandibular dystonia: Speech effects. In C. Moore, K. Yorkston, & D. Beukelman (Eds.), *Dysarthria and apraxia of speech: Perspectives on management* (pp. 227–241). Baltimore: Paul H. Brookes Publishing Co.

Scientific Advisory Board of the Dystonia Medical Research Foundation. (1988). Cited in S. Fahn, C. Marsden, & D. Calne (Eds.), *Advances in neurology: Vol. 50. Dystonia 2.* New York: Raven Press.

Chapter 5

Aerodynamic Evaluation of Parkinsonian Dysarthria
Laryngeal and Supralaryngeal Manifestations

L. Carol Gracco, Vincent L. Gracco,
Anders Löfqvist, and Kenneth P. Marek

THE SPEECH OF individuals with Parkinson's disease (PD) is characterized by reduced stress, increased rate, monotonic pitch, loudness, and imprecise consonant production (Darley, Aronson, & Brown, 1975). Acoustically, such speech has decreased duration of voiced segments, reduced fundamental frequency variations, and limited formant trajectories at consonant-vowel transitions as compared to normal, age-matched controls (Canter, 1967; Darley et al., 1975; Forrest, Weismer, & Turner, 1989; Logeman, Fisher, & Boshes, 1978; Ludlow, Bassich, Connor, Coulter, & Lee, 1987; Ludlow & Schulz, 1989; Ramig, Scherer, Titze, & Ringel, 1988; Weismer, 1983). Although specific and detailed analyses of parkinsonian deficits have been limited, existing studies of laryngeal and supralaryngeal structures suggest that the reduction in intelligibility characteristic of Parkinson's disease may be a result of manifestations of this disorder throughout the entire vocal tract musculature. For example, studies of lip and jaw movements have reported reduced amplitude and veloc-

This work was supported in part by NIH Grant No. DC-00044, DC-00594, DC-00865, and DC-00121 from the National Institute of Deafness and Other Communication Disorders. This work is in the public domain.

65

ity (Caligiuri, 1987; Connor, Abbs, Cole, & Gracco, 1989) and a cinegraphic study of laryngeal kinematics in PD (Hanson, Gerratt, & Ward, 1984) revealed a correlation between abnormalities in the phonatory posture of laryngeal structures and voicing deficits. These manifestations may involve the control and coordination of laryngeal and supralaryngeal events. Taken together, these factors result in overall reduction in speech intelligibility in individuals with PD. Hence, the simultaneous evaluation of upper articulator and laryngeal dynamics may give a more complete analysis of deficit behaviors that ultimately influence intelligibility.

The perceptual significance of aerodynamic events and the utility of aerodynamic measures as a basis for understanding speech and voice articulation have been known for some time. With few exceptions, however, attempts to associate complex articulatory and phonatory changes with time-varying changes in supraglottal air pressure and airflow have been rare. Much of the basic and applied literature investigating pressure and flow parameters has focused on differences in peak amplitude as a function of a variable such as vocal intensity, place, and manner of production, or has used peak amplitude to provide measures of glottal resistance. In isolation, peak measures are little more than a description of system output, providing limited information regarding the underlying articulatory dynamics.

In a clinical setting, procedures that sample both temporal aspects of laryngeal and supralaryngeal dynamics as well as peak measures associated with various speech motor disorders are regarded as time consuming. This study provides the basis for a relatively easy and efficient evaluation of laryngeal and supralaryngeal articulation in individuals with parkinsonian dysarthria. The methodology is based on work by Müller and Brown (1980) and Gracco and Miller (1981), which illustrates the significance of assessing time-varying pressure and flow characteristics. Müller and Brown focused on description of aerodynamic features associated with voiced and voiceless bilabial consonants. In the present study, steady-state airflow rates for vowels were also measured, making the estimation of vocal tract resistance possible. Thus, laryngeal articulatory gestures are considered along with upper articulator events to interpret the effects of specific movement disorders on vocal tract dynamics.

METHODS

Subjects

The salient speech characteristics and demographic data for five adult subjects are summarized in Tables 1 and 2. Three subjects (JC, HM, and AB) had symptoms involving the speech production mechanism and all

Table 1. Summary of speech characteristics for five subjects with Parkinson's disease

Subjects	Speech characteristics
JH	• Minimal reduction in intelligibility • Mildly breathy vocal quality • Accurate consonant production with infrequent alterations of speech rate
AD	• Minimal reduction in intelligibility • Mildly breathy vocal quality • Accurate consonant production with infrequent alterations of speech rate
HM	• Minimal reduction in intelligibility • Hoarse and breathy vocal quality • Accurate consonant production with occasional alterations of speech rate
AB	• Moderately to severely impaired intelligibility • Reduced vocal intensity • Imprecise consonant production • Accelerated speech rate
JC	• Moderately to severely impaired intelligibility • Reduced vocal intensity • Imprecise consonant production • Inappropriately slowed speech rate

extremities. These subjects, each on high and frequent dosages of Sinemet, were characterized as having severe bradykinesia, masked faces bilaterally, and pronounced cogwheel rigidity with tremor. Speech intelligibility was moderate to severely impaired in both female subjects, (JC and AB), characterized by reduced intensity, imprecise consonant production, and inappropriately slowed or accelerated speech rate. Subject HM showed minimal reduction in speech intelligibility despite the severity of symptoms in the limbs. Vocal quality was characterized as hoarse and breathy, with accurate consonant production and occasional alteration of speech rate. The two remaining subjects, (JH and AD) were mildly impaired, with mild symptoms specific to one upper extremity that were well controlled on low dosages of Sinemet. Vocal quality for these two subjects was characterized as mildly hoarse and breathy.

Table 2. Demographic data

Subjects	Sex	Age	Duration PD	H/Y[a]	UPDRS[b]
AD	M	74	2	1	19
JM	M	60	5	2.5	38
AB	F	50	10	4	82
HM	M	50	13	4	79
JC	F	49	22	4	93

[a]Hoehn and Yahr (H/Y).
[b]United Parkinson's Disease Rating Scale (UPDRS).

Tasks

Three tasks were consistently performed within 1 hour post-medication. First, subjects were instructed to produce a vowel-consonant-vowel (VCV) disyllable with V being /æ/ or /i/ and C being /p/ or /b/. Ten repetitions of each disyllable were obtained at a comfortable speaking rate. Each of the ten disyllables were produced after a single breath. Subjects were instructed to breathe as they would in any normal speaking situation. Second, four repetitions of the sustained vowel /a/ of four-second length were acquired at conversational pitch and intensity levels. Third, seven consecutive repetitions of the syllable /pæ/ at the same requested pitch and intensity levels were obtained in single trials.

Equipment

Aerodynamic signals were obtained using a Rothenberg mask equipped with transducers to sense airflow at the mouth (Microswitch model 163) and air pressure in the oral cavity (Microswitch model 162). A short (approximately 10 cm) polyethylene tube, placed in the oral cavity behind the lips, was used to sense the pressure associated with bilabial closure. The acoustic signal was transduced with a microphone at a distance of approximately 15 cm from the subjects' lips. All signals were digitized at 5000 Hz with 12-bit resolution. Once acquired, filtered versions of the pressure and flow waveforms were generated and stored as separate files for analysis. The pressure and airflow signals were software-filtered at 80 Hz prior to calculating the measures reported below.

Measures

Laryngeal/Supralaryngeal Timing   As illustrated in Figure 1, both amplitude and temporal measures were extracted from the disyllable sequences. They are defined as follows: 1) T_c—duration of the closing phase, defined as the time difference between the initial registration of air pressure (P_o) and the associated timing of minimum airflow; 2) T_r— duration of the opening or consanant release phase, defined as the time between the onset of the pressure drop (at release) and the return of pressure to baseline. In addition, peak intraoral pressure (P_p) and peak airflow (P_u) at the instant of release were obtained.

Mean Flow Rate/Laryngeal Resistance   Aerodynamic measures were used to evaluate changes in the physiological state of the vocal folds during sustained phonation. One consequence of glottic insufficiency or inadequate closure of the glottis is greater than normal mean airflow rate (MFR) (Hirano, 1981; Isshiki & von Leden, 1964; Iwata, von Leden, & Williams, 1972; Shigemori, 1977; Yoshioka, Sawashima, Hirose, Ushijima, & Honda, 1977). MFR was based on an averaged 50 msec sample

GRAPHIC SUMMARY OF MEASUREMENT SCHEME

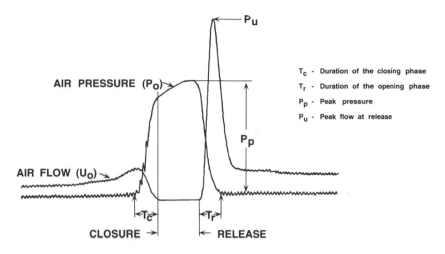

Figure 1. A summary of the measurement scheme employed for the analysis of the time-varying pressure/flow variations.

from the mid-portion of the sustained vowel /a/. In addition, laryngeal resistance (defined as the ratio of subglottal pressure to average subglottal air flow) was estimated from simultaneous measures of airflow and intraoral air pressure during repetitions of the syllable /pæ/ based on the method outlined by Smitheran and Hixon, 1981.

RESULTS

A number of laryngeal and supralaryngeal sequelae were observed in varying degrees in the five subjects. Although intersubject variability was high, intrasubject variability was generally low. Each subject presented a consistent set of behaviors across repetitions and across tasks.

Amplitude Measures/Pressure and Flow

Figures 2 and 3 summarize the peak intraoral air pressure and peak airflow during bilabial consonant production for the five subjects. All subjects demonstrate a voiced/voiceless difference with voiceless pressures and air flow higher than their voiced counterparts. Peak intraoral air pressure for the voiced and voiceless bilabials ranged from 6 to 8 cm H_2O for /p/ and 2 to 5 cm H_2O for /b/. With the exception of peak pressure for the voiced bilabial for subject AB (2 cm H_2O), these values are within the range of normal speakers (Subtelney, Worth, & Sakuda, 1966). Peak flow rates ranged from 100 to 1180 ml/sec for /p/ and 40 to 550 ml/sec for /b/.

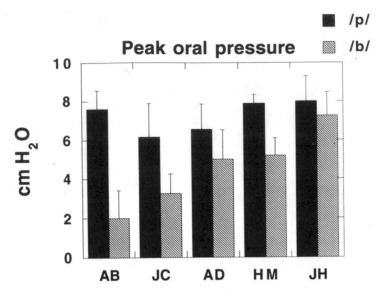

Figure 2. Peak intraoral air pressure (cm H₂O) for consonant production of /p/ and /b/ for five subjects.

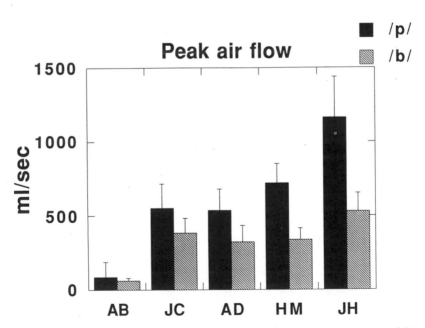

Figure 3. Peak airflow (ml/sec) for the five subjects for the stop consonant productions /p/ and /b/.

Again, with the exception of the flow rates for subject AB, these values are within the normative range (Gilbert, 1973; Isshiki & Ringel, 1964).

Mean flow rates obtained during the mid-portion of the vowels /a/ and /i/ varied for the different subjects. Flow rates for Subject HM were essentially normal, ranging from 150 to 250 ml/sec during the steady-state portion of the vowels. Flow rates for subjects JC, AB, and AD were quite variable, ranging from 40 to 100 ml/sec. Given the presence of adequate peak intraoral pressures, it can be assumed that the respiratory driving force was not the major contributor to the reduced flow. Rather, mean flow rates suggest elevated resistance to air flow.

In support of this interpretation were the estimates of laryngeal resistance. Figure 4 represents the mean flow rates, peak intraoral pressure, and derived laryngeal resistance measures obtained during /pæ/ repetitions. In general, the laryngeal resistance values obtained were higher than those reported for normal subjects (Hillman, Holmberg, Perkell, Walsh, & Vaughn, 1989; Smitheran & Hixon, 1981) and ranged from 20 to 58 cmH$_2$O/L/sec for the five subjects. Figure 5 shows examples from seven serial repetitions of /pæ/ for subjects HM and AB illustrating the extremes. Laryngeal resistance for this sample for subject HM was calculated at 30 cmH$_2$O/L/sec. As can be seen, flow rates averaged approximately 250 ml/sec and pressures ranged from 7.4 to 9.2 cm H$_2$O. A distinct voiceless interval can be seen during the closure based on the airflow signal. In contrast, laryngeal resistance values for subject AB were much higher, averaging almost 60 cmH$_2$O/L/sec. Peak pressures are much more variable and decline rapidly over the course of the series of repetitions. It can also be seen that flow rates are extremely low, averaging approximately 60 ml/sec. Interestingly, it seems that, as articulation continues, voicing becomes continuous, and voiceless /p/ becomes the voiced cognate /b/. This is possibly due to increased laryngeal resistance or glottal spasm. It can also be seen that repetition rate for subject AB increases over the 5-second interval, consistent with her tendency toward acceleration.

Temporal Measures/Pressure and Flow Variations

Figure 6 is a summary of the duration of the closing phase (T$_c$) for the lips during voiced and voiceless consonants /p/ and /b/. This value reflects a portion of the change in cross-sectional area at the lips during the oral closing for the stop. The horizontal line in the graph is the average value for this variable reported by Müller and Brown (1980). There was a tendency for all subjects, with the exception of JH, to display significantly longer values than those obtained from normal subjects. These values reflect, in part, overall rate of articulation; that is, slow oral closing movements can result in higher T$_c$ values. Of the five subjects in the present

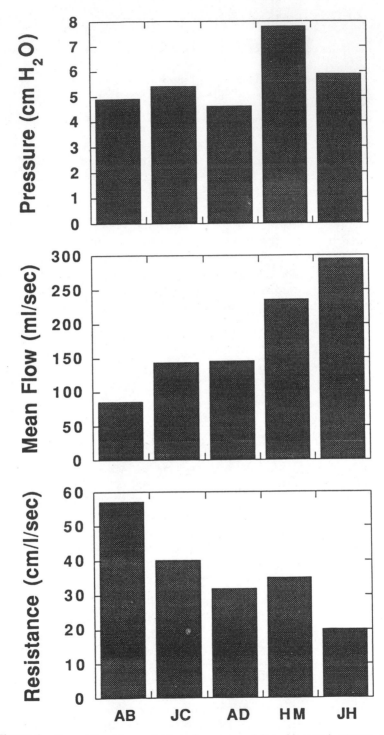

Figure 4. Mean airflow rates, peak intraoral pressure, and derived laryngeal resistance measures obtained during /pæ/ repetitions.

/pae/ Repetitions

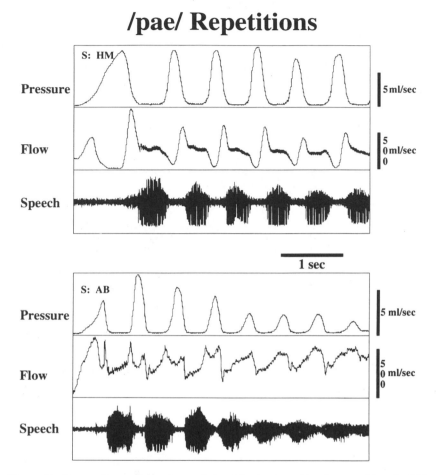

Figure 5. Pressure, flow, and acoustic speech signals for /pæ/ repetitions for two subjects. For HM /p/ closures are all associated with laryngeal devoicing, whereas AB tends to continue voicing into the voiceless consonant after two repetitions.

study, subjects HM, AD, and JH display normal speaking rates. Subjects JC and AB display slowed speaking rates and associated slowed lip and jaw movements. Although the rate of speech of subject AB was decreased, this rate reduction was not as dramatic as that of subject JC. In this case, it would not be expected to see greater T_c values for subject AB as compared to JC. Inspection of the pressure/flow waveforms from subject AB reveal the reason for the longer T_c values. For most of her VCV productions, complete cessation of air flow was not achieved, apparently due to velar insufficiency. As such, T_c values reflect a combination of the closing interval and a portion of the occluded phase of stop consonant production. As noted previously, subject JC also demonstrated apparent velar insufficien-

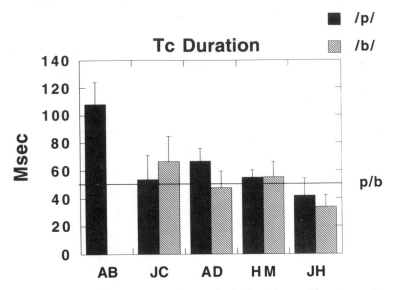

Figure 6. Mean duration of the closing phase (T$_c$) for the five subjects collapsed across the two vowels. No significant vowel affects were noted (p > .05). Data from subject AB illustrate no data because zero flow was not apparent. Horizontal line indicates the average T$_c$ values for /p/ and /b/ reported by Müller and Brown (1980).

cy, but to a lesser degree than AB. In this case, occlusion was apparent from the rapid decrease in oral airflow.

Figure 7 is a summary of the results for the duration of the release phase (T$_r$); the horizontal lines reflect the average T$_r$ values for voiceless /p/ and voiced /b/ from Müller and Brown (1980). For the T$_r$ measure for the voiceless /p/, all subjects displayed lower mean values than those reported by Müller and Brown. It should be noted that the range for the five subjects reported in Müller and Brown for /p/ was approximately 100–220 msec. Although the values in this present study may fall on the low side of the normal range, it should be noted that for voiceless stops, the presence of an expiratory breath pulse will lengthen T$_r$ and that, under normal conditions, an expiratory breath pulse is necessary to produce T$_r$ values greater than 150 msec (Müller & Brown, 1980). The short T$_r$ values in our study suggest that none of the subjects with dysarthria in this study generated an expiratory breath pulse coincident with oral release.

One of the most consistent findings by Müller and Brown (1980) was a longer T$_r$ interval for voiceless compared to voiced stops. In the present investigation this was true for only three of the five subjects. Subjects AB and JC displayed longer than normal durations for the time required for the pressure to return to baseline (T$_r$) following oral release of the voiced consonant. Time for release is influenced by any variable that can influ-

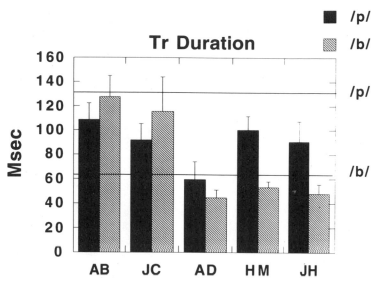

Figure 7. Mean duration of the release phase (T$_r$) for the five subjects collapsed across the two vowels. No significant vowel effects were noted (p > .05). Horizontal lines indicate the average T$_r$ values reported by Müller and Brown (1980) for /p/ and /b/.

ence the time constant of the decay rate of the air pressure. According to Fant (1960) and Stevens (1956), the following factors may explain the longer T$_r$ durations for the voiced stops for AB and JC: 1) slower oral release gesture, or 2) large air volumes in the subglottal and supraglottal cavities coupled with decreased resistance at the glottis due to an incomplete closure. If the lower peak pressures for /b/ compared to /p/ can be used as an indication of laryngeal approximation (hence adequate glottal resistance), then the most plausible explanation for the longer T$_r$ values for the voiced stops is a slowed release gesture at the point of oral articulation.

As suggested above, in the absence of kinematic data, simultaneous examination of pressure/flow interactions can be used to infer laryngeal/supralaryngeal coordination and timing. As shown in Figure 1, normal subjects show a reduction in airflow as bilabial occlusion occurs for /p/. In addition, voicing usually ceases in coordination with lip contact and glottal open. Abnormal patterns are noted for the two of the five subjects presented in Figure 8. For AB, complete devoicing was not observed. The flow pattern in conjunction with the continuation of voicing, identified by the arrows, shows evidence of incoordination in oral/laryngeal timing. That is to say, there is evidence in the speech signal that the glottis did not open, or from the flow signal that the lips did not close completely. Laryngeal devoicing begins much earlier than oral closing, as evidenced

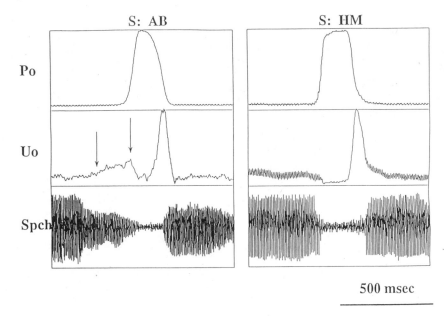

S: AB

S: HM

Po

Uo

Spch

500 msec

Figure 8. Pressure, flow, and acoustic signals for /æpæ/ illustrating examples of the T_c measure for subjects AB and HM.

by the increase in flow noted by the arrows. In contrast, HM displays a decrease in flow and a rather abrupt cessation in voicing at the moment of pressure rise as the lip area decreases to the minimum value to reflect pressure change. In the case of AB, oral/laryngeal actions were observed to be discoordinated or slowed. For HM, however the transition was closer to normal, although accelerated.

DISCUSSION

This study is an initial investigation of vocal tract deficits in a group of individuals with Parkinson's disease based in part on previous work by Müller and Brown (1980). A variety of laryngeal and supralaryngeal impairments were noted. For three of the five subjects, vocal tract resistance fell within a range consistent with normal speakers. Limb symptoms in these subjects were mild. Measured vocal tract resistance was high in one subject. This may reflect excessive muscle tension at either the level of the glottis or supraglottis. At the least, however, it represents vocal tract constriction. In this subject, vocal tract behavior was consistent with symptoms of muscular rigidity in the limbs. For another subject, however, limb symptoms did not seem to predict vocal tract findings. Subject HM had moderate-to-severe limb involvement; the lower limbs were more severely impaired than the upper limbs, and the upper limbs were more impaired than the bulbar musculature. Vocal tract resistance and glottal/supraglottal timing measures were essentially normal.

Supralaryngeal differences were noted in two of the five subjects. Inferences from the time-varying pressure/flow waveforms suggested that oral closing and opening movements were slowed, a finding consistent with previous speech movement studies. In addition, there was some indication of laryngeal/supralaryngeal discoordination.

From this limited sample it is possible to suggest, but not to confirm, that laryngeal or vocal tract resistance measures may be useful to document a variety of perceptual voice characteristics previously reported for individuals with PD. However, the speech symptoms may not always correlate or correspond to those of the limbs. The time-varying characteristics of the supraglottal pressure and flow waveforms are the consequence of the concomitant articulatory events associated with stop consonant production. Simultaneous recordings and analysis of the pressure and flow events may become easily obtained indicators of global system performance, thus aiding in diagnosis of certain speech-related disorders and providing insight into the abnormal articulatory process. For example, the T_r measure or duration of the release phase is defined as the time between the onset of airflow and return to baseline. All the subjects, with possibly one exception, showed short T_r values for the voiceless /p/. This measure reflects not only the release gesture at the point of articulation, but any variable that can influence the time constant of the decay rate of air pressure. In the present context, the short T_r values for /p/ may reflect a rapid devoicing gesture, perhaps coupled with discoordination of the lips and larynx. For the two most severely involved subjects (AB and JC), the T_r durations for the voiceless /b/ were longer than normal, suggesting elevated laryngeal/vocal tract resistance, a slowed release gesture, or the presence of an expiratory breath pulse. Given the low peak pressure values for these subjects, excessive vocal tract resistance seems the most plausible conclusion.

It is especially important to consider that these measures did differentiate subjects within a group of individuals with parkinsonian dysarthria. Just as there exist subgroups of patients with Parkinson's disease and various subgroups of Parkinson's syndrome, it seems that acoustic/perceptual and aerodynamic data may be useful in differentiating these populations further. Additionally, pressure and flow information can aid in identifying laryngeal manifestations of pathophysiology affecting phonatory characteristics and glottal efficiency. The preceding dynamic analysis scheme can be used to provide specific information on the general functioning of the speech production mechanism, as well as interarticulatory timing from an objective set of data. An analysis scheme of this type in conjunction with acoustic and perceptual performance indices, may generate more informed hypotheses concerning the nature of the underlying motor deficit(s) as they affect the speech mechanism.

REFERENCES

Caligiuri, M.P. (1987). Speech labial kinematics in parkinsonian rigidity. *Brain, 110*, 1033–1044.

Canter, G.J. (1967). Neuromotor pathologies of speech. *American Journal of Physical Medicine, 46*, 659–666.

Connor, N.P., Abbs, J.H., Cole, K.J., & Gracco, V.L. (1989). Parkinsonian deficits in serial multiarticulate movements for speech. *Brain, 112*, 997–1009.

Darley, F.L., Aronson, A.E., & Brown, J.R. (1975). *Motor speech disorders.* Philadelphia: W.B. Saunders.

Fant, G. (1960). *Acoustic theory of speech production.* The Hague: Moulton and Co.

Forrest, K., Weismer, G., & Turner, G.S. (1989). Kinematic, acoustic, and perceptual analyses of connected speech produced by Parkinsonian and normal geriatric adults. *Journal of the Acoustical Society of America, 85*, 2608–2622.

Gilbert, H.R. (1973). Oral airflow during stop consonant production. *Folia Phoniatrica, 25*, 288–301.

Gracco, V.L., & Miller, E.M. (1901). *Analysis of supraglottal air pressure variations in spastic dysarthria.* Paper presented at the 1981 Convention of the American Speech-Language-Hearing Association, Los Angeles, CA.

Hanson, D.G., Gerratt, B.R., & Ward, P.H. (1984). Cinegraphic observations of laryngeal dysfunction in Parkinson's disease. *Laryngoscope, 94*, 348–353.

Hillman, R.E., Holmberg, E.B., Perkell, J.S., Walsh, M., & Vaughan, C. (1989). Objective assessment of vocal hyperfunction: An experimental framework and initial results. *Journal of Speech and Hearing Research, 33*, 373–392.

Hirano, M. (1981). *Clinical examination of voice.* New York: Springer-Verlag.

Holmberg, E.B., Hillman, R.E., & Perkell, J.S. (1988). Glottal airflow and transglottal air pressure measurements for male and female speakers in soft, normal, and loud voice. *Journal of the Acoustical Society of America, 84*, 511–529.

Isshiki, N., & Ringel, R. (1964). Air flow during the production of selected consonants. *Journal of Speech and Hearing Research, 7*, 233–244.

Isshiki, N., & von Leden, H. (1964). Hoarseness aerodynamic studies. *Archives of Otolarynology—Head and Neck Surgery, 80*, 206–213.

Iwata, S., von Leden, H., & Williams, D. (1972). Air flow measurement during phonation. *Journal of Communication Disorders, 5*, 67–79.

Logeman, J.A., Fisher, H.B., & Boshes, B. (1978). Frequency and co-occurrence of vocal tract dysfunction in the speech of a large sample of Parkinson's patients. *Journal of Speech and Hearing Disorders, 43*, (1) 47–57.

Ludlow, C.L., Bassich, C.J., Connor, N.P., Coulter, D.C., & Lee, Y.J. (1987). The validity of using phonatory jitter and shimmer to detect laryngeal pathology. In T. Baer, C. Sasaki, & K. Harris (Eds.), *Laryngeal function in phonation and respiration* (pp. 463–474). Boston: Little, Brown.

Ludlow, C.L., & Schulz, G.M. (1989). Stop consonant production in isolated and repeated syllables in Parkinson's disease. *Neuropsychologia, 27*, 829–838.

Müller, E.M., & Brown, W.S. (1980). Variations in the supraglottal air pressure waveform and their articulatory interpretation. In N. Lass (Ed.), *Speech and language: Advances in basic research and practice* (Vol. 4). New York: Academic Press.

Ramig, L.A., Scherer, R.C., Titze, I.R., & Ringel, S.P. (1988). Acoustic analysis of voice patients with neurological disease: Rationale and preliminary data. *Annals of Otology, Rhinology and Laryngology, 97,* 164–171.

Shigemori, Y. (1977). Some tests related to the air usage during phonation. Clinical investigations. *Otologia Fukuoka—Jibi to Rinsho, 23,* 138–166.

Smitheran, J.R., & Hixon, T.J. (1981). A clinical method for estimating laryngeal airway resistance during vowel production. *Journal of Speech and Hearing Disorders, 46,* 138–146.

Stevens, K. (1956). Stop consonants. *Massachusetts Institute of Technology. Research Laboratory of Electronics. RLE Progress Report.* 198–213.

Subtelney, J.D., Worth, J.H., & Sakuda, M. (1966). Intraoral pressure and rate of flow during speech. *Journal of Speech and Hearing Research, 9,* 498–518.

Weismer, G. (1983). *Acoustic descriptions of dysarthric speech: Perceptual correlates and physiological inferences.* Speech Motor Control Laboratories Progress Report. Madison, WI: Wasiman Center.

Yoshioka, H., Sawashima, M., Hirose, H., Ushijima, T., & Honda, K. (1977). Clinical evaluation of air usage during phonation. *Japanese Journal of Logopedics and Phoniatrics, 18,* 87–93.

Chapter 6

Vowel Variability in Developmental Apraxia of Speech

Beverly Smith, Thomas P. Marquardt,
Michael P. Cannito, and Barbara L. Davis

DEVELOPMENTAL APRAXIA OF speech (DAS) is a neurologically based disorder affecting the ability to program movements for speech volitionally in the absence of impaired neuromuscular function. Although the disorder has been defined in similar terms for more than 30 years, there is little agreement about its most salient characteristics or the most appropriate assessment and treatment regimens (Guyette & Diedrich, 1981; Marquardt & Sussman, 1991).

DAS typically is included within a broader syndrome marked by delayed expressive language, impaired nonverbal oral movements, and reduced performance on tests of verbal intelligence (Marquardt & Sussman, 1991). Prominent speech characteristics include reduced diadochokinetic rates, high frequency of omission errors, additional errors on later developing speech sounds, frequent vowel errors, increased errors on longer utterances, prosodic abnormalities, and inconsistent speech errors. Guyette and Diedrich (1981) argued, however, that there was: 1) little agreement on the behaviors or symptoms necessary for diagnosis; 2) little empirical evidence to support conclusions, even when agreement was found; and 3) no precise description of how these data could be used as diagnostic indicators of DAS. This chapter investigates a frequently cited feature of DAS, articulatory variability in vowel production, to determine if it is a salient characteristic of the disorder.

Anecdotal reports of vowel errors are frequently reported in studies of DAS. Rosenbek and Wertz (1972) noted that misarticulations of children with DAS include vowel errors of substitution and distortion. Crary (1984) reported that 23 of 25 children with DAS used the phonological process of vowel neutralization. However, the average strength (ratio of occurrence to opportunity) of vowel neutralization was only 5%. Love and Fitzgerald (1984) found that their 7-year-old subject with DAS produced 8% vowel errors on single words and five percent on sentences, but Yoss and Darley (1974) reported that vowel errors did not discriminate between children divided into groups on the basis of performance on a task of isolated, volitional oral movements. Pollock and Hall (1989) provided a systematic description of vowel errors in five children with DAS. They found that vowel errors were not random but followed common patterns including laxing, backing, lowering, tensing, and diphthong reduction. These results suggest that vowel errors may be an important feature of DAS, but the results are inconclusive.

A similar lack of agreement is seen relative to articulatory consistency in DAS. Yoss and Darley (1974) and Smartt, LaLance, Gray, and Hibbett (1974) did not find evidence that children with DAS were more inconsistent than children with functional articulation disorders. Bowman, Parsons, and Morris (1984), in a phonological process analysis study of data from Williams, Ingham, and Rosenthal (1981), concluded that children with DAS were consistent as a function of type of processes used and effects of performance load. Schumacher, McNeil, Vetter, and Yoder (1986) analyzed three consecutive repetitions of 20 stimuli from elicited word, imitated word, and imitated sentences from 15 children divided into those with DAS, nonapraxic phonological impairment, and normal children, and reached a different conclusion. Based on analysis of variability scores derived from repeated productions, they concluded that children with DAS were significantly more variable than were children with phonologic delay and normal children.

In this investigation, acoustic analyses of vowel productions were undertaken to examine articulatory variability in a child with DAS, children with articulation delayed, and normal children.

METHOD

Subjects

Three males from 8 years to 8 years and 10 months served as subjects. One subject demonstrated developmental apraxia of speech and was matched on the basis of age with a child demonstrating a nonapraxic phonologic/articulation deficit and with a child with normal speech and language skills. The subjects, from monolingual English-speaking families, demonstrated normal auditory acuity bilaterally based on pure tone audiometric screening at 500, 1000, 2000, 4000, and 6000 Hz, and normal speech structures based on results from the Oral Speech Mechanism Screening Examination (St. Louis & Ruscello, 1981).

Results from the Templin-Darley Test of Articulation (TDAT) (Templin & Darley, 1969), the Test of Auditory Comprehension of Language–Revised (TACL–R) (Carrow-Woolfolk, 1985), and the Peabody Picture Vocabulary Test–Revised (PPVT) (Dunn & Dunn, 1981) were used to assign the children to the diagnostic categories. The subject with developmental apraxia had been followed for 2 years. His speech production was characterized by a severe articulation disorder, simple syllable shapes, inconsistent articulation errors, and marked difficulty on longer utterances. On the TDAT, sounds in error included /r/, /ð/, θ/, /ʒ/, and /j/. In blends, /w/ was substituted for /r/. Other cluster errors included /lk/, /kt/, and /pt/. Administration of the Screening Test for Developmental Apraxia of Speech (Blakeley, 1980) at age 6 years and 9 months yielded a weighted score of −369, which was interpreted as a 99% probability of correct assignment to an apraxia of speech diagnostic category. Diagnosis of developmental apraxia was based on findings of normal receptive language (TACL % = 32), difficulty sequencing oral movements, a severe articulation disorder (TDAT score = 98), reduced expressive language, and cognitive ability within normal limits based on previous testing.

The subject with nonapraxic articulation delay demonstrated normal language development (TACL % = 45) with an articulation test score more than one standard deviation below the mean for his age (TDAT score = 121). Error sounds on the TDAT included substitutions for /s/ and /z/. The normal subject demonstrated speech (TDAT score = 141) and language development (TACL % = 32) within one standard deviation of the mean for his age.

Stimuli

The subjects imitated a series of stimuli within three conditions. Task 1 included 10 isolated vowels (i, I, e, æ, ɛ, u, ʊ, o, ɔ, a) produced 10 times in random order. Task 2 was comprised of the same vowels produced five times in randomized order in g-vowel-g, d-vowel-d, g-vowel-d, and d-vowel-g consonant-vowel-consonant (CVC) contexts. Task 3 contained a series of consonant-vowel-consonant-vowel (CVCV) nonsense syllables divided into four groups on the basis of syllable transition difficulty. The first group included four reduplicated nonsense words (e.g., /baba/). The second group required movement for vowels from high front to low back tongue position (e.g., /babi/). The third and fourth groups included identical vowels in varying contexts (e.g., /puzu/) and more complex tongue movements for the production of consonants and vowels (e.g., /gaku/). Task 3 stimuli were produced five times in random order.

Procedures

The subjects were seated in a sound attenuated booth approximately six inches from a Sony external microphone, model F-105. Productions were recorded on a Marantz professional cassette recorder, model PMD 220. For each task, the subject was required to imitate the stimulus presented by the examiner. If the subject did not produce the intended vowel target(s), the stimulus was re-presented to ensure that perceptually unambiguous vowel productions were available for analysis. This procedure was continued until the full complement of responses was obtained from each subject for each of the three tasks. Rest periods were provided after each task in order to maintain attention and reduce fatigue.

Data Analysis

Each child produced a total of 100 isolated vowels, 200 consonant-vowel-consonant (CVC) sequences, and 80 CVCV sequences. The stimuli were analyzed using MacSpeech Lab II, version 1.0 (GW Instruments, Inc., 1988). Each production was digitized for visual inspection, and the first and second formants of the vowel were identified. Measurements of formant frequencies were obtained at the vowel steady-state center and at points approximately 40 msec after the beginning and 40 msec before the termination of the vowel steady state. Formants 1 and 2 were determined from the Linear Predictive Coding (LPC) plot (sampling rate 10 kHz). If necessary to resolve ambiguity from the LPC spectra, a Fast Fourier Transform (FFT) plot also was utilized in the decision-making process. The three measurements were averaged to obtain the frequency of each formant. Vowel durations also were obtained for the CVC and CVCV stimuli.

RESULTS

First formant (F1) and second formant (F2) frequency means and standard deviations were determined for each vowel and were used to compute mean coefficients of variation (mean/standard deviation) for each subject and task. Similarly, duration means and standard deviations were used to compute mean coefficients of variation for the vowels in the one- and two-syllable task conditions.

F1 variability for the three subjects in isolation, CVC, and CVCV contexts is shown in Figure 1. Average coefficients of variation were comparable for the child with articulation delay and the normal subject. They ranged from 0.095 (isolation) to 0.130 (CVCV context) for the subject with articulation delay and from 0.093 (CVCV context) to 0.101 (CVC context) for the normal child. In contrast, coefficients for the child with DAS ranged from 0.222 for isolation to 0.249 for the CVCV context. For

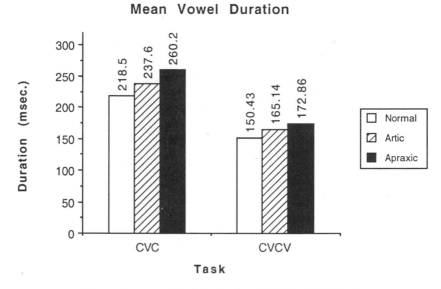

Mean Vowel Duration

Figure 1. F1 variability for isolated vowel, CVC, and CVCV tasks.

each context, coefficients for the subject with apraxia were twice as large as for the subject with articulation delay and the normal subject.

F2 variability is shown in Figure 2. Coefficients of variation for the subject with articulation delay and the nondisabled subject were comparable for the isolation (articulation delayed = 0.107; normal = 0.084), CVC (articulation delayed = 0.118; normal = 0.127) and CVCV (articulation delayed = 0.096; normal = 0.114) contexts. The coefficients for the subject with apraxia, however, were almost two times greater (isolation, 0.209; CVC, 0.224; CVCV, 0.227) than for the other two subjects.

Two vowels were examined to determine the number of productions of F1 within two standard deviations of the mean based on data from Syrdal and Gopal (1986). A large proportion of the F1 values of the subject with apraxia were more than two standard deviations from the mean. For the vowel /æ/, for example, F1 values of the subject with apraxia were within two standard deviations for 54% of the productions compared to 80% for the subject with articulation delay and 100% for the normal subject.

Mean CVC and CVCV vowel durations are shown in Figure 3. Vowel durations were greater for CVC productions than for CVCV. Durations were shortest for the normal subject (CVC = 218.5 msec; CVCV = 150.43 msec) followed by the subject with articulation delay (237.6 msec; 165.14 msec) and the subject with apraxia (260.2 msec; 172.86 msec).

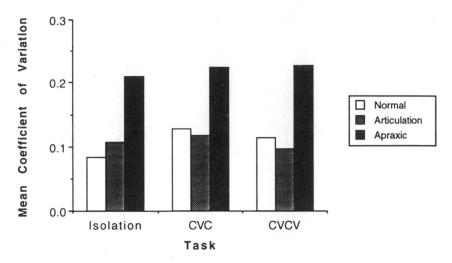

Figure 2. F2 variability for isolated vowel, CVC, and CVCV tasks.

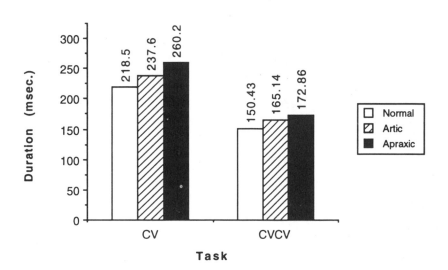

Figure 3. Mean vowel duration for CVC and CVCV tasks.

Figure 4 shows the duration mean coefficients of variation for the three subjects. Coefficients were similar for the CVC stimuli. However, coefficients were greater for the subject with apraxia (0.280) compared to the subject with articulation delay (0.246) and normal subjects (0.223) for the CVCV stimuli. These results suggest that the subject with apraxia was more variable on durational measures of vowel production for two syllable stimuli.

DISCUSSION

Previous studies of articulatory consistency in developmental apraxia of speech have been based primarily on phonetic and phonological process analyses. For example, Bowman et al. (1984) found that children with DAS were consistent as a function of type and frequency of phonological processes used. In contrast, Schumacher et al. (1986) analyzed three consecutive productions of 20 stimuli from elicited word, imitated word, and imitated sentence conditions and found that children with apraxia were less consistent than nonapraxic phonologically delayed and normal children, based on a matching analysis of repeated productions. Marquardt and Sussman (1991) reported preliminary data that suggested that the incidence of substitution and omission errors varies as a function of stimulus length and that a child with DAS may demonstrate a high frequency of changes in production of phonetic elements in words.

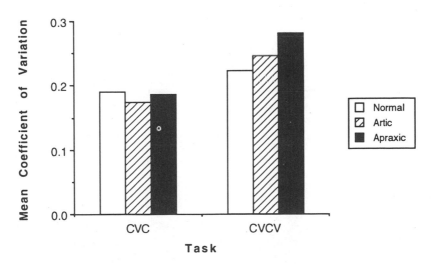

Figure 4. Vowel duration variability for CVC and CVCV tasks.

Acoustic analyses provide a more fine-grained analysis of articulatory consistency. The results of this study, although preliminary because they are based on only one child with DAS, suggest that these children are more variable, particularly in the frequency domain. Formant frequencies were more variable for the subject with DAS than for the subject with articulation delay and the normal child, and durational variability was greater on two-syllable productions.

A speculative, neural-based theory to account for increased variability in DAS was proposed by Marquardt and Sussman (1991). They argued that the underlying etiology of DAS is the lack of neural substrates responsible for phonemic identification and categorization that must concurrently develop with speech motor output skills. Deficits in skilled motor articulations can be viewed as stemming from a deficient internal target representation of the phonemic elements needed to guide the motor output algorithms of speech production. A deficient target representation system for phonemic elements would have the effect of producing multiple off-target productions to target phones. Increased vowel variability would be expected to be one feature of the deficient targeting system.

REFERENCES

Blakeley, R.W. (1980). *Screening test for developmental apraxia of speech.* Tigard, OR: C.C. Publications, Inc.

Bowman, S.N., Parsons, C.L., & Morris, D.A. (1984). Inconsistency of phonological errors in developmental verbal dyspraxic children as a factor of linguistic task and performance load. *Australian Journal of Human Communication Disorders, 12,* 1090–1191.

Carrow-Woolfolk, E. (1985). *Test for auditory comprehension of language-revised.* McAllen, TX: DLM Teaching Resources.

Crary, M.A. (1984). Phonological characteristics of developmental verbal dyspraxia. *Seminars in Speech and Language, 5,* 71–82.

Dunn, L.M., & Dunn, L.M. (1981). *Peabody Picture Vocabulary Test—Revised.* Circle Pines, MN: American Guidance Service.

Guyette, T.W., & Diedrich, W.M. (1981). A critical review of developmental apraxia of speech. In N.J. Lass (Ed.), *Speech and language: Advances in basic research and practice* (Vol. 5). New York: Academic Press.

Love, R.J., & Fitzgerald, M. (1984). Is the diagnosis of developmental apraxia of speech valid? *Australian Journal of Human Communication Disorders, 12,* 71–82.

Marquardt, T.P., & Sussman, H.M. (1991). Developmental apraxia of speech: Theory and practice. In D. Vogel & M. Cannito (Eds.), *Disordered speech motor control.* Austin, TX: PRO-ED.

Pollack, K.E., & Hall, P.K. (1989). *An analysis of the vowel misarticulations of five developmentally apraxic children.* Paper presented at the Convention of the American Speech-Language-Hearing Association, St. Louis, MO.

Rosenbek, J., & Wertz, R.T. (1972). A review of fifty cases of developmental apraxia of speech. *Language, Speech and Hearing Services in Schools, 3,* 23–33.

Schumacher, J.G., McNeil, M.R., Vetter, D.K., & Yoder, D.E. (1986). *Journal of the Acoustical Society of America*. Paper presented at the Convention of the American Speech-Language-Hearing Association, New Orleans, LA.

Smartt, J., LaLance, L., Gray, J., & Hibbitt, P. (1976). Tennessee Speech and Hearing Association subcommittee report. *Journal of the Tennessee Speech and Hearing Association, 20*, 21–39.

St. Louis, K.O., & Ruscello, D.M. (1981). *Oral speech mechanism screening examination*. Baltimore: University Park Press.

Syrdal, A.K., & Gopal, H.S. (1986). A perceptual model of vowel recognition based on the auditory representation of American English vowels. *Journal of the Acoustical Society of America*, 1086–1100.

Templin, M.C., & Darley, F.L. (1969). *Templin-Darley Test of Articulation*. Iowa City: IA: University of Iowa.

Williams, R., Ingham, R.J., & Rosenthal, J. (1981). A further analysis for developmental apraxia of speech in children with defective articulation. *Journal of Speech and Hearing Research, 24*, 496–505.

Yoss, K.A., & Darley, F.L. (1974). Developmental apraxia of speech in children with defective articulation. *Journal of Speech and Hearing Research, 17*, 399–415.

Chapter 7

Diadochokinesis for Complex Trisyllables in Individuals with Spasmodic Dysphonia and Nondisabled Subjects

Michael P. Cannito, Pinar Ege,
Farhan Ahmed, and Steven Wagner

ALTHOUGH SPASMODIC OR spastic dysphonia (SD) historically has been viewed as a hyperfunctional voice disorder of psychogenic origin (Arnold, 1959), in recent years researchers have come to regard SD as a focal adventitious movement disorder related to dystonia or essential tremor, or both (Aminoff, Dedo, & Izdebski, 1978; Aronson, Brown, Litin, & Pearson, 1968; Aronson & Hartman, 1981; Blitzer, Lovelace, Brin, Fahn, & Fink, 1985; Ludlow & Connor, 1987; Rosenfield, 1988). The finding of a high incidence of abnormal extrapyramidal motor signs external to the larynx in this population supports this claim (Cannito, Kondraske, & Johns, 1991). A particular category of motor dysfunction that has been noted in SD is the reduction of the patient's ability to execute rapid, alternating movements of speech and nonspeech structures, resulting in dysdiadochokinesia or slow, irregular, alternating movement rates (Aronson et al., 1968; Cannito & Kondraske, 1990; Cannito et al., 1991; Pool et al., 1991).

A recent study by Pool et al. (1991) reported abnormal, rapid, alternating movement rates as the most prominent finding of neurologic examinations of 45 SD subjects. Almost half the sample exhibited some abnormalities of rate or rhythm in the lower extremities, upper extremities, or tongue. Instrumental quantification of abnormal, rapid, sequential movements in SD has also been provided. Cannito and Kondraske (1990) observed a significant reduction in speed for complex sequential movements of the upper extremities for 18 patients with SD in the presence of normal manual reaction times, relative to matched nondisabled controls. Cannito et al. (1991) similarly reported slower than normal diadochokinetic rates for the production of complex syllable sequences in the same 18 subjects with SD and the nondisabled control subjects. They produced repetitive tokens of the trisyllable /tukipa/ as rapidly as possible, using a whisper voice to minimize the effects of laryngospasms on speech production. A significant moderate Pearson product moment correlation was observed between the speech-sequencing task and the dominant hand pegboard performance in the SD group ($r = .524$; $df = 16$; $p < .05$) that did not exist in the controls ($r = .084$; $df = 16$; $p > .10$). These findings seem to support a generalized deficit for rapid, complex, voluntary movement sequencing in at least some patients with SD. In addition to the diadochokinetic abnormalities, there have been persistent reports of articulatory difficulties in patients with SD, despite the fact that the voice problem remains the most salient presenting symptom (see Cannito, 1989). This chapter explores the nature of abnormal diadochokinesis in individuals with SD further by providing a fine-grained acoustical evaluation of temporal characteristics of rapidly articulated, reiterant conditions that might interact with normal and disordered vocal motor control. Specifically, it was of interest to determine whether individuals with SD and normal subjects would perform differently on all voiced, voiced–voiceless, and whispered sequences, and whether adductor versus abductor subtypes of SD could be differentiated on the basis of voicing contrasts. Clinically derived a priori expectations were that subjects with adductor SD would have greater difficulty with all voiced sequences, subjects with abductor SD with voiced–voiceless sequences, and that both subtypes would perform better on whispered than on phonated productions (Cannito, 1986).

Although maximum performance tests of syllable repetition rate have been criticized as unrepresentative of natural speech (Kent, Kent, & Rosenbeck, 1987; Tiffany, 1980), they do provide some estimate of the upper limits of coordinative serial movement function. Quantitative acoustic measurements derived from tasks of this type have been shown to be sensitive to differences between normal speakers with dysarthria, and between subtypes of speakers with dysarthria (Portnoy & Aronson, 1982; Tatsumi, Sasanuma, Hirose, & Kiritani, 1979). The issue is that the task should be viewed as a specialized test of motor function, as it is in the neurologic examination, rather than as an evaluation of speaking ability. Considering the particular difficulty that subjects with SD seem to exhibit on diadochokinetic and related rapid sequencing tasks, further investigation of the phenomenon in this population is warranted.

METHODS

Subjects

Experimental subjects were 10 females with spasmodic dysphonia who had been diagnosed by at least two speech-language pathologists and an otolaryngologist familiar with the disorder. At the time of experimental testing, each subject was submitted to an in-depth voice evaluation to ensure adherence to diagnostic criteria detailed in Cannito and Kondraske (1990). Five subjects exhibited adductor SD characterized by voice stoppage with intermittent strain-strangled voice quality, and five exhibited abductor SD characterized by voice stoppage with intermittent breathiness. None had undergone recurrent laryngeal nerve resection or botulinum toxin injection. All had received some speech therapy, but with no lasting relief of SD symptoms. Ten nondysphonic and otherwise nondisabled control subjects were matched to the subjects with SD by age, gender, and handedness. All subjects were monolingual English speakers without complicating histories of neurologic, psychiatric, or communication disorders. Characteristics of the subjects with SD are provided in Table 1.

Procedures

The experimental task consisted of each subject producing an eight reiterant trisyllable sequence of /dugiba/ (voiced), /tukipa/ (voiced-voiceless), and /tukipa/ (whispered) as rapidly as possible. The reiterant paradigm is useful because it strips away the confounding influence of assimilation from coarticulating segments and reduces linguistic processing demands (Kelso, Vatikiotis-Bateson, Saltzman, & Kay, 1985; Tiffany, 1980). The

Table 1. Spasmodic dysphonic subject characteristics

Subject number	Type of spasm	Voice tremor	Dysphonic severity	Age in years
1	ADductor	+	Mild	50.17
2	ADductor	−	Profound	62.00
3	ADductor	−	Profound	65.10
4	ADductor	+	Moderate	64.17
5	ADductor	+	Moderate	55.42
6	ABductor	+	Moderate	61.67
7	ABductor	−	Severe	42.58
8	ABductor	−	Moderate	28.92
9	ABductor	+	Mild	46.58
10	ABductor	+	Moderate	37.10

particular phonetic sequences were selected to increase the front-to-back complexity of serial movement requirements for articulation of both the vowels and consonants. Contrastive voicing conditions were incorporated to provide differential glottal opening and closing requirements that might interact with laryngospasm types.

Three acceptable trials were elicited in each of three voicing conditions. An acceptable trial was one in which the requested phonemic sequence /dugiba/, /tukipa/, or /tukipa/ was produced in a perceptually accurate manner without phonemic errors, respiration pauses, or dysfluency. Accuracy was judged on line by the examiner, a certified speech-language pathologist experienced with individuals with neurologic impairment. Subjects were instructed specifically to "Say _____ as rapidly as you can, but don't go so fast that you say the wrong thing." In some cases, trials from both individuals with SD and control subjects were aborted because subjects were using articulatory imprecision (e.g., spirantization of consonants, vowel neutralization, or voicing assimilation) as a strategy to increase speed. The problem of speed versus accuracy tradeoffs in diadochokinesis has been addressed by Luschei (1991).

Speech samples were recorded in a single-walled IAC Model 400A sound-isolated booth where the subject was seated comfortably with her head supported in an adjustable Ritter dental chair. Subject's speech was recorded using a head-worn Countryman® EM-101 electret condensor microphone (positioned approximately 8 cm from the left corner of the subject's mouth) and a Countryman® EM-101 preamplifier. The preamplifier was connected to an Otari 5050 reel-to-reel recorder. Recorded signals were subsequently digitized at 10 kHz samples/sec with a 4.5 kHz anti-aliasing filter. Acoustic analyses consisted of a series of duration measures completed using the G. W. Instruments MacSpeech Lab II (Downey, Hancock, Hemme, & Weinreb, 1988) software and hardware implemented on a Macintosh II computer. Temporal measurements were obtained via moveable vertical cursors with simultaneous wide-band spectrogram and waveform displayed on the CRT. The experimental measures included:

1. Individual trisyllable durations, measured from the onset of burst noise for the initial alveolar stop to the offset of glottal pulsing for the terminal /a/of each trisyllable (This yielded eight trisyllable durations per trial, with three trials per voicing condition = 72 trisyllable durations per subject.)
2. Inter-trisyllable transition durations, measured from the offset of terminal /a/ to the onset of burst noise for the subsequent alveolar stop for each trisyllable (This yielded seven transition durations per trial, with three trials per voicing condition = 63 transition durations per

subject.) Coefficients of variation (cov = standard deviation divided by the mean) were then computed for each eight trisyllable sequence to provide an index of variability within a repetition series for

3. Trisyllable durations
4. Inter-trisyllable transitions (These represented an index of irregularity of the alternating motion rate.)
5. Total articulation time (sum of eight trisyllable durations)
6. Total transition time (sum of seven transition durations) was also computed. As an additional accuracy check, the total sequence durations were measured independently and determined to agree within 10 ms with the sum of the total articulation and total transition times for every sequence.

To establish reliability of measurement procedures, two judges independently completed all measures of the same samples for 30% of the data from both subject groups. Inter-rater reliability coefficients for all measures were computed separately for subjects with SD and control subjects and exceeded $r = .95$ ($p < .001$) in every case.

Four-factor repeated measures analyses of variance (ANOVAs) (groups × voicing conditions × trials × repetitions) were computed for the variables of trisyllable duration and inter-trisyllable transitions. In each ANOVA, individual repetitions within an eight trisyllable train constituted the repeated measure. This dimension was included in the design to explore possible systematic alterations of duration across a repetition train. For example, festination might appear as a progressive decrease across repetitions, whereas muscle fatigue might appear as a progressive increase. Simple one-way ANOVAs were also computed to compare performance of individuals with adductor and abductor SD and normal controls on the variables of total articulation time, total transition time, and for the coefficients of variation of articulation time and transition time for individual repetition trains. Post hoc means comparisons were performed using Tukey's Honestly Significant Difference test at alpha level .05 (Winer, 1977).

RESULTS

Descriptive statistics were computed for both the group with SD and the control group for the temporal variables of total duration, articulation time, and inter-trisyllable transition time, as well as coefficients of variation for trisyllable durations and inter-trisyllable transitions. These are shown for each voicing condition in Table 2.

A four-factor, repeated measures ANOVA (groups × voicing conditions × trials × repetitions) was computed for individual trisyllable dura-

Table 2. Means and standard deviations for temporal variables for subjects with spasmodic dysphonia and normal subjects, by voicing condition

Variable	Group	Voiced	Voiced–voiceless	Whispered
Total speaking time	NC	5.286 (0.408)[a]	4.750 (0.313)	4.761 (0.295)
	SD	5.867 (1.038)	5.740 (0.840)	5.518 (0.869)
Total articulation time	NC	4.417 (0.256)	4.073 (0.376)	4.045 (0.354)
	SD	4.916 (0.854)	4.899 (0.692)	4.766 (0.776)
Total transition time	NC	0.850 (0.316)	0.679 (0.184)	0.716 (0.209)
	SD	0.914 (0.536)	0.830 (0.470)	0.754 (0.225)
COV[b] trisyllable durations	NC	0.039 (0.019)	0.046 (0.017)	0.039 (0.013)
	SD	0.049 (0.024)	0.079 (0.057)	0.060 (0.037)
COV intertrisyllable transitions	NC	0.139 (0.094)	0.112 (0.054)	0.091 (0.037)
	SD	0.187 (0.151)	0.198 (0.198)	0.188 (0.185)

NC = normal control subjects; SD = subjects with spasmodic dysphonia.
[a]Means are followed by standard deviations in parentheses.
[b]COV = coefficient of variation.

tions. Significant main effects of groups ($F = 57.86$, $df = 1,162$; $p = .0001$) and voicing conditions ($F = 3.09$; $df = 2,162$; $p = .0483$) were observed. Subjects with SD exhibited significantly longer trisyllable durations than nondisabled controls. Trisyllable durations in the voiced condition were longer than those in either the voiced-voiceless or whispered conditions ($p < .05$) for both groups. No other main or interaction effects achieved statistical significance.

A four-factor ANOVA (groups × voicing conditions × trials × repetitions) was computed for inter-trisyllable transition durations. A statistically significant main effect of repetitions was observed ($F = 15.14$; $df = 6,972$; $p = .0001$) as was a significant groups × repetitions interaction ($F = 3.41$; $df = 6,972$; $p = .0025$). Whereas both groups exhibited a progressive lengthening of transitions across the trisyllable sequences, analysis of simple effects demonstrated that the increased transition durations were only statistically significant within the group with SD ($F = 9.81$; $df = 6,1074$; $p = .0001$). This interaction is depicted graphically in Figure 1. No other effects achieved statistical significance.

Comparisons between the groups with adductor and abductor SD were performed using simple one-way ANOVAs. For total articulation time, there was a significant between-group effect ($F = 36.52$; $df = 2,179$; $p = .0001$). Post hoc tests ($p < .05$) indicated that the mean for the group with adductor SD was significantly longer than that of the mean for the group with abductor SD, and that both subtypes were significantly greater than the controls. For total transition time, there was also a significant between-group effect ($F = 13.17$; $df = 1,179$; $p = .0001$). Post hoc tests indicated that the mean for the group with adductor SD was significantly longer than that of either the group with abductor SD or the nondisabled

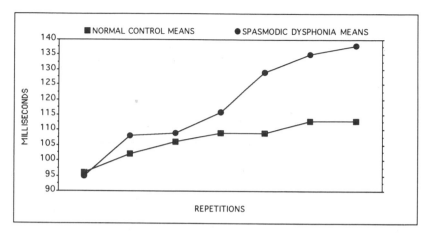

Figure 1. The groups × repetitions interaction for inter-trisyllable transition durations, illustrating progressive lengthening by the subjects with spasmodic dysphonia.

control group, who did not differ from each other. (See Figures 2 and 3.)

Significant between-group effects were also observed for coefficients of variation of trisyllable durations ($F = 10.94$; $df = 2,179$; $p = .0001$) and inter-trisyllable transitions ($F = 9.14$; $df = 2,179$; $p = .0002$). For trisyllable durations, both subgroups with abductor and adductor SD demonstrated significantly ($p < .05$) greater variability than the controls, but did not differ from each other. For inter-trisyllable durations, only the subgroup with adductor SD was significantly more variable than the nondisabled control group.

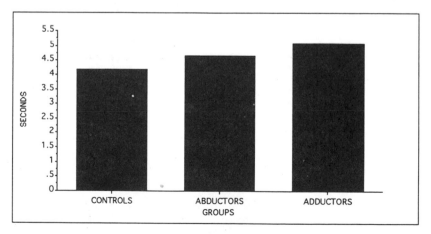

Figure 2. Mean total articulation time per eight repetition sequence for subgroups with spasmodic dysphonia and normal controls.

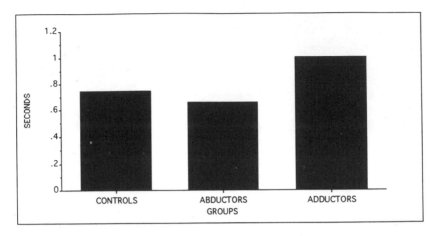

Figure 3. Mean total transition time per eight repetition sequence for subgroups with spasmodic dysphonia and normal controls.

DISCUSSION

Temporal acoustic analyses of the diadochokinetic utterances employed in this study yielded a number of relevant findings. First, the measurement technique was highly reliable and demonstrated sensitivity to the phonetic contrast between voiced and voiceless syllable productions. One plausible explanation for the increased trisyllable durations noted in the all-voiced condition is the allophonic constraint on vowel lengthening preceding voiced stops in English (Ladefoged, 1982). This rule was apparently observed by both the subjects with SD and the nondisabled subjects to a similar degree.

Subjects with SD generally exhibited longer and more variable trisyllable durations across voicing conditions than did control subjects. This is consistent with earlier reports of diadochokinetic abnormalities in individuals with SD. Contrary to expectations, however, the subjects with SD did not demonstrate more normal repetition rates when whispering. Also contrary to expectations was the lack of differentiation of the groups with adductor and abductor SD on the basis of voicing contrasts. These results may suggest a disassociation of voice quality per se and articulatory sequencing ability in individuals with SD. It is possible that subjects with adductor and abductor SD may be differentiated on the basis of voice quality ratings of all voiced versus voiced–voiceless or whispered utterances, although their diadochokinetic rates on these materials were similar. This question should be investigated further, because it raises the possibility of co-occurring phonatory and articulatory deficits as opposed to merely a lack of coordination between phonatory and articulatory activity in individuals with SD, as proposed by Aronson et al. (1968).

Interestingly, subgroups with adductor and abductor SD were differentiated from each other on dimensions other than voicing contrasts. Both types of subjects with SD evidenced abnormally slow and irregular trisyllable articulation; however, the subjects with adductor SD were substantially slower than were those with abductor SD. In addition, those with adductor SD exhibited abnormally slow and irregular inter-trisyllable transitions not present in those with abductor SD. One possible explanation for these findings is that patients with adductor SD may have a generalized slowing and fragmentation of speech production, whereas patients with abductor SD may have difficulty with a particular aspect of consonant-vowel (CV) syllable articulation, such as voice onset time. This hypothesis is currently being investigated in our laboratory.

In conclusion, acoustical analyses of the diadochokinetic utterances employed in this study were sensitive to differences among individuals with adductor or abductor SD and nondisabled controls, and also to the phonetic contrast of voicing. This may have been due to the emphasis placed on phonetic accuracy—in addition to speed—during data elicitation. The demand for correct production should have resulted in a task more difficult than one that required speed alone. As a result, subjects may have slowed their rate of production in order to achieve the specified targets. The added complexity of a vowel sequence, representing extreme places of articulation in lieu of neutral vowels used in previous research, combined with the stop consonant sequence, may also have enhanced diagnostic sensitivity.

The results of this study concur with previous findings of Portnoy and Aronson (1982) and Tatsumi et al. (1979) that acoustical diadochokinetic measures are not only sensitive to differences between speakers with motor speech disorders and nondisabled speakers but also to differences among subgroups within the larger group with motor speech disorders. Thus, despite criticisms of diadochokinetic measures in the literature, it is suggested that arguments for or against the utility of such measures in motor speech assessment and research still remain unresolved.

REFERENCES

Aminoff, M.J., Dedo, H.H., & Izdebski, K. (1978). Clinical aspects of spasmodic dysphonia. *Journal of Neurology, Neurosurgery and Psychiatry, 41*, 361–365.

Arnold, G.E. (1959). Changing interpretations of a persistent afflication. *Logos, 2,* 3–14.

Aronson, A.E., Brown, J.R., Litin, M.E., & Pearson, J.S. (1968). Spastic dysphonia: Voice neurologic and psychiatric aspects. *Journal of Speech and Hearing Disorders, 33,* 203–218.

Aronson, A.E., & Hartman, D. (1981). Adductor spastic dysphonia as a sign of essential (voice) tremor. *Journal of Speech and Hearing Disorders, 46,* 52–58.

Blitzer, A., Lovelace, R.E., Brin, M.F., Fahn, S., & Fink, M.E. (1985). Electro-myographic findings in focal laryngeal dystonia (spastic dysphonia). *Annals of Otology, Rhinology and Laryngology, 94*, 591–594.

Cannito, M.P. (1986). Speech diadochokinesis and spasmodic dysphonia: A clinical note. *Texas Journal of Audiology and Speech Pathology, 12*, 25.

Cannito, M.P. (1989). Vocal tract steadiness in spasmodic dysphonia. In K.M. Yorkston & D.R. Beukelman (Eds.), *Recent advances in clinical dysarthria* (pp. 243–262). Boston: Little, Brown.

Cannito, M.P., & Kondraske, G.V. (1990). Rapid manual abilities in spasmodic dysphonic and normal female subjects. *Journal of Speech and Hearing Research, 33*, 123–133.

Cannito, M.P., Kondraske, G.V., & Johns, D.F. (1991). Oral-facial sensorimotor function in spasmodic dysphonia. In C.A. Moore, K.M. Yorkston, & D.R. Beukelman (Eds.), *Dysarthria and apraxia of speech: Perspectives on management* (205–225). Baltimore: Paul H. Brookes Publishing Co.

Downey, A., Hancock, R., Hemme, K., & Weinreb, G. (1988). *MacSpeech lab II users manual.* Sommerville, MA: G.W. Instruments.

Kelso, J.A.S., Vatikiotis-Bateson, E., Saltzman, E.L., & Kay, B. (1985). A qualitative dynamic analysis of reiterant speech production: Phase portraits, kinematics, and dynamic modeling. *Journal of the Acoustical Society of America, 77*, 266–280.

Kent, R.D., Kent, J.F., & Rosenbeck, J.C. (1987). Maximum performance tests of speech production. *Journal of Speech and Hearing Disorders, 52*, 367–387.

Ladefoged, P. (1982). *A course in phonetics.* San Diego: Harcourt Brace Jovanovich.

Ludlow, C., & Connor, N. (1987). Dynamic aspects of phonatory control in spasmodic dysphonia. *Journal of Speech and Hearing Research, 30*, 197–206.

Luschei, E.S. (1991). Development of objective standards of nonspeech oral strength and performance: An advocates view. In C.A. Moore, K.M. Yorkston, & D.R. Beukelman (Eds.), *Dysarthria and apraxia of speech: Perspectives on management* (pp. 3–14). Baltimore: Paul H. Brookes Publishing Co.

Pool, K.D., Freeman, F.J., Finitzo, T., Hayashi, M., Chapman, S.B., Devous, M.D., Close, L.G., Kondraske, G.V., Mendelsohn, D., Schaefer, S.D., & Watson, B.C. (1991). Heterogeneity in spasmodic dysphonia: Neurologic and voice findings. *Archives of Neurology, 48*, 305–309.

Portnoy, R.A., & Aronson, A.E. (1982). Diadochokinetic syllable rate and regularity in normal and in spastic and ataxic dysarthric subjects. *Journal of Speech and Hearing Disorders, 47*, 324–328.

Rosenfield, D.B. (1988). Spasmodic dysphonia. In J. Jankovic & E. Tolosa (Eds.), *Advances in neurology, Vol. 49. Facial dyskinesias* (pp. 317–327). New York: Raven Press.

Tatsumi, I.F., Sasanuma, S., Hirose, H., & Kiritani, S. (1979). Acoustic properties of ataxic and Parkinsonian speech in syllable repetition tasks. *Annual Bulletin of the Royal Institute of Logopedics and Phoniatrics* (Tokyo), *13*, 99–104.

Tiffany, W.R. (1980). The effects of syllable structure on diadochokinetic and reading rates. *Journal of Speech and Hearing Research, 23*, 894–908.

Winer, B.J. (1971). *Statistical principles in experimental design.* New York: McGraw-Hill.

ADVANCES IN DIAGNOSTIC ASSESSMENT

Chapter 8

Application of Instrumental Techniques in the Assessment of Dysarthria
A Case Study

Carl A. Coelho, Vincent L. Gracco, Marios Fourakis, Maria Rossetti, and Kiyoshi Oshima

THE TRADITIONAL APPROACH to the assessment of dysarthria has been, and in most clinical settings continues to be, based upon auditory perceptual judgments including measures of articulatory accuracy (Enderby, 1983), speech intelligibility (Yorkston & Beukelman, 1981), or subjective ratings of specific speech dimensions (e.g., phonation, resonance, articulation) (Darley, Aronson, & Brown, 1975). Although a variety of objective instrumental measures (e.g., EMG, kinematics, aerodynamic, acoustic) is currently available for delineating the physiology of speech production, to date, clinical application of these techniques has been limited (Gerratt, Till, Rosenbek, Wertz, & Boysen, 1991). It has been argued that the lack of widespread clinical use of instrumental measures in the management of dysarthria is because such measures are indirect and their predictive value has not been established (McNeil, 1986). Other explanations include the lack of instrumentation in most clinical settings and clinicians' limited understanding of the relevancy of instrumentally acquired data to patient management. In other words, many clinicians tend to use those measures that are available and with which they are most comfortable. Generally, these have been perceptual measures.

Yorkston, Beukelman, and Bell (1988) note that because dysarthria is typically associated with disease processes or chronic conditions management of the communication deficits of individuals with dysarthria must be functionally oriented and compensatory, as opposed to being directed toward a return to normalcy. Development of an effective individualized treatment program requires an understanding of the components underlying normal speech as well as the impact of pathologies on these processes. This goal is consistent with what Netsell, Lotz, and Barlow (1989) have identified as the primary purpose of a clinical speech physiology examination.

Addition of instrumental measures to the assessment of dysarthria secondary to closed head injury (CHI) would seem to be clinically advantageous. The nature of these dysarthrias has been poorly documented because few studies have been undertaken (Yorkston et al., 1988). In addition, because the mechanism of injury in CHI often results in both focal and diffuse brain damage, the resulting patterns of deficits may be quite complex and confusing.

This chapter describes the application of a variety of instrumental measures to the assessment of speech production in a young female, 5 years post onset of a CHI. Data obtained from instrumental and perceptual measures during various speech tasks are compared and discussed with regard to differential diagnosis, identification of compensatory mechanisms, and treatment planning.

METHOD

Subject

The subject, RB, is a 36-year-old right-handed female who was a college graduate and a captain in the army when she suffered a closed head injury in a fall during jump school training at a military installation. CT scan at the time of injury revealed a right subdural hematoma and blood in the fourth ventricle. Neurologic work-up noted RB to have a diffuse cerebral injury as well as injury to her left basal ganglia and cerebellum with resulting right hemiparesis. Generalized slowness of movement consistent with damage to the basal ganglia produced a parkinsonian-like complex of symptoms.

RB's communicative impairments included relatively mild cognitive deficits and a moderate-to-severe hypokinetic dysarthria. Her dysarthria was characterized by reduced loudness and stress, monopitch, breathiness, inconsistent articulatory undershooting and spirantization, and speech produced in short rapid bursts. Initially, RB also demonstrated a severe dysphagia with primary difficulty noted in the oral stage of the swallow.

At the time of testing, RB was approximately 5 years post onset of CHI. She had been actively involved in both in- and outpatient rehabilitation programs since her injury and continued to receive periodic physical and speech therapy, as well as taking singing lessons. Her dysarthria at that time was rated as mild. Scores on the Assessment of Intelligibility of Dysarthric Speech (AIDS) (Yorkston & Beukelman, 1981) were 94% for single words (transcription format) and 98% for sentences. Speaking rate was approximately 122 words per minute and her efficiency ratio (intelligible words per minute/190) was 0.63. Swallowing function was within normal limits.

Instrumental Analysis

Instrumental analysis was carried out at Haskins Laboratories. Two-dimensional movements (inferior–superior, anterior–posterior) of the upper lip, lower lip, and jaw were obtained using a standard optoelectronic device. Small light-emitting diodes (LEDs) were placed on the upper and lower lip vermillion borders in the midsagittal plane; jaw motion was obtained from a LED placed on the external extension of a custom-fitted jaw splint providing direct transduction of jaw movement uncontaminated by skin movement. Air pressure within the vocal tract was sensed using a Millar pressure transducer (SPC-350) inserted transnasally and located during recording within the oropharynx. The subject's acoustic signal was transduced with a Sennheiser (MKH816T) microphone placed at a distance of 5 cm from her mouth.

Movement characteristics of the upper articulators were evaluated during a number of speech and nonspeech tasks, including jaw opening and closing, lip pursing and retracting, repetition of /u–i/, /sæ/, and /pæ/ at normal and maximally fast rates (RB was instructed to produce each utterance several times at a normal rate and then several times "as fast as you can"), the production of single words in carrier sentences, and repetition of short bilabially loaded sentence material. Quantitative evaluation focused on the frequency of repetitive productions, maximum displacements of the respective articulators and their velocities, overall speaking rate, segmental durations, and relative timing among articulators during bilabial production. From the aerodynamic recordings, the magnitude of intraoral pressures for various sounds, as well as pressure rise and fall times, were obtained.

Acoustic Analysis

Acoustic recordings were done at Gaylord Hospital. A list of target words containing the nine pure vowels of American English in the context of [b_d], and the three front vowels in the context [C_d], where C was one of the following [b,d,g]. The list also contained the following six words, "pap," "pab," "tap," "tab," "cap," "cab." The target words were embedded in two carrier sentences, either "Today, the password is XXXX," or "Today, XXXX is the password," where "XXXX" was the target. Two repetitions of each word in each carrier sentence comprised two lists, which were randomized separately. RB was recorded reading these lists while seated in an audiology testing booth in front of an AKG C-451EB/CK-1 microphone-preamplifier combination. The utterances were recorded onto a SONY-75ES digital audio tape recorder, running in 16-bit mode at 20-kHz sampling rate. After the recording each utterance was digitized and stored on a Macintosh IIci computer, using the commercially available Sound Design II software package, using 16-bit resolution and 22-kHz sampling rate. At digitization time, the utterances were normalized for amplitude. Each utterance was then processed using the commercially available software package *Signalyze* (Keller, 1990) and the following measurements were made.

The first two formants of each vowel in the [b_d] context were measured at approximately one third through the vowel duration, from a 1024-point Fast Fourier transform-derived spectrum. Using the same spectral analysis setup, measurements of the first two formants of the three vowels [i, e, æ] after [b,d,g] were taken at 10-ms intervals starting at vowel onset and continuing up to 90 ms into the vowel. These values were used to graph the formant transitions out of the target initial consonants for each vowel. Temporal measurements were made directly from the waveform, as displayed on a high-resolution monitor and they included: initial consonant closure, voice onset time (if any), vowel duration, and final consonant closure.

RESULTS

The results from the speech movement and aerodynamic measures are presented first followed by those from the acoustic analyses. The quantitative results for each movement task focused on the major axis of motion for the relevant articulator or articulators. For example, measurement of lip pursing and retraction and /u–i/ repetition focused on upper and lower lip movements in the anterior–posterior dimension; jaw opening and closing, /pæ/, and /sæ/ repetitions focused on movements in the inferior–superior direction.

Repetitive Movements

Overall, RB's frequency of movement repetition was found to be slowed for both the speech (syllable repetition) and nonspeech tasks (purse/retract lips and open/close jaw). Because all articulators moved at essentially the same rate for each of the various conditions, results are not articulator specific. Her repetition rates ranged from 0.7 to 1.8 movement cycles per second for /u–i/, /pa/, /wa/, and /sa/ (see Figure 1). Her nonspeech rates were slower than the speech repetitions, ranging from 0.3 to 0.8 cycles per second for lip pursing/retracting and jaw opening/closing, respectively. Although no norms are available for nonspeech repetitive movements, norms for syllable repetitions measured acoustically should be directly comparable. As such, RB's repetition rates are considered slower than normal (see Baken, 1987, for a summary of results from various investigations). RB's maximally fast productions generally increased by a factor of two for all tasks. In addition to RB's overall slowed rate, her movement displacements and velocities for the repetitive tasks were found to be reduced as well, most notably in the upper and lower lips (see Figure 2). For example, during the repetitive syllables /sæ/ and /pæ/, her jaw displacements ranged from 8.0 to 10.0 mm respectively. In contrast, her lower lip displacement for the /pæ/ repetitions ranged from 2.5

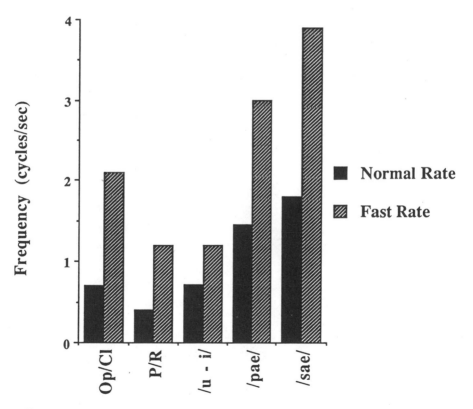

Figure 1. RB's movement repetition rates for speech (syllable repetition) and nonspeech (purse/retract lips and open/close jaw) tasks.

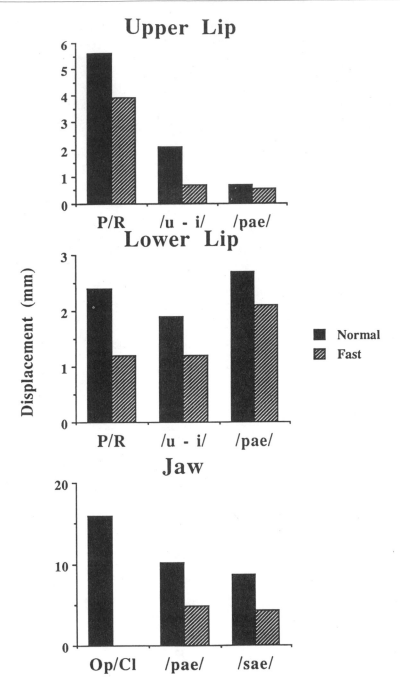

Figure 2. RB's movement displacements for speech (syllable repetition) and nonspeech (purse/retract lips and open/close jaw) tasks.

to 3.0 mm. RB's lower lip velocity was also found to be reduced from normal. As shown in Figure 3, RB's lower lip closing velocities (at the bottom left) were extremely low, ranging from 20 to 30 mm/sec. Her jaw opening and closing velocities were higher and within the normal range. Overall, RB's movement displacements and velocities of her upper and lower lips for the different repetitive tasks were reduced, while those of her jaw were within or close to the normal range. When rate was increased, lip movements became most undetectable, particularly for her upper lip.

The differential degree of impairment in RB's lips compared to her jaw was also noted during production of single word and sentence material. Figure 4 depicts a comparison of the inferior–superior lower lip and jaw movement for the word "suffer" produced in the carrier sentence "It's a suffer again" by RB and a normal control subject. The jaw movement for the two subjects provides an interesting comparison. For RB, the jaw opening displacement was reduced for the vowel, whereas the jaw closing displacement contributed significantly more to the achievement of the /f/ constriction. The lower lip movement for the constriction was reduced for RB compared to the normal subject. In addition to slowed rate and reduced movement displacement and velocity, there were other indications of impaired lip movement.

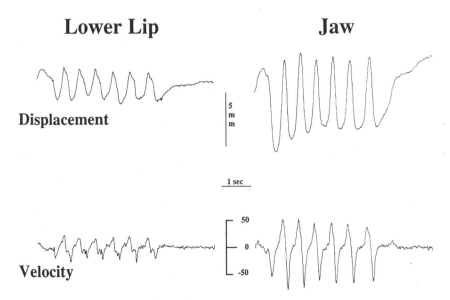

Figure 3. Comparison of RB's movement displacements and velocities for her lower lip and jaw during repetitions of /pæ/.

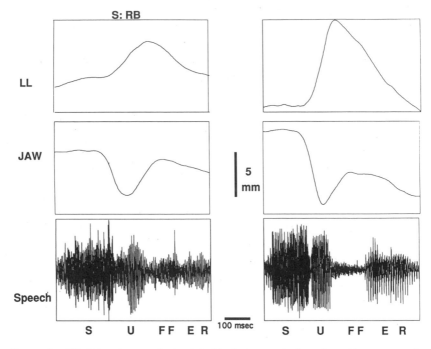

Figure 4. RB's (left) and a normal subject's (right) inferior–superior lower lip and jaw movement for the word "suffer" produced in the carrier sentence "It's a suffer again."

Figure 5 is a single example of RB's anterior–posterior movements of the upper and lower lips during alternating repetitions of the vowels /u/–/i/. Again, although no norms were available for the extent of the movement displacements, it can be seen that the two lips were not moving smoothly. Although the upper and lower lips were generally moving at the same time, the movement displacements were small, approximately 1–3 mm with evidence of a high frequency (around 8 Hz) tremor. Finally, RB's sentence length utterances exhibited a large degree of token-to-token variability, more so than is observed with normal speakers.

Aerodynamic assessment indicated that RB's peak pressures were generally within normal limits, although her flow rates were always greater than normal, often as high as 400 cc/sec. During production of verb-consonant-verbs (VCVs) where V was /æ/ or /i/ and C was /p/ or /b/, simultaneous measures of peak oral pressure and airflow were obtained. Figure 6 is a single example of the flow and pressure relations for /æpæ/. The peak pressure at /p/ closure was approximately 8 cm of water with peak flow at lip release of approximately 600 cc/sec, both well within normal limits. Flow rate averaged over a half-second period during the vowel resulted in a flow rate during the vowel of approximately 390 cc/sec.

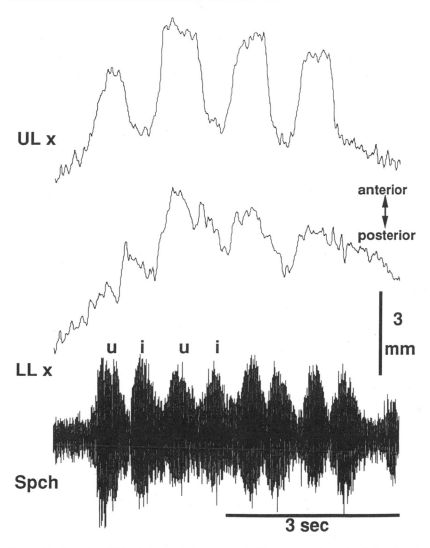

Figure 5. Example of RB's anterior–posterior movements of the upper and lower lips during alternating repetitions of the vowels /u/–/i/.

The high flow rate is consistent with the perceived breathy quality of her voice and fiberoptic examination of the larynx confirmed that RB had incomplete vocal cord approximation. Pulmonary function testing also indicated that RB's lung volumes and flow rates were within normal limits. It seemed that the reduced respiratory support suggested from perceptual analysis was rather a reflection of adequate respiratory support coupled with inefficient laryngeal valving.

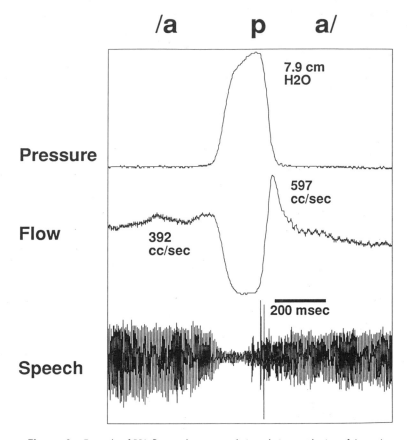

Figure 6. Example of RB's flow and pressure relations during production of /æpæ/.

Acoustics

The mean frequencies of RB's first and second formants are plotted in Figure 7, along with the mean frequencies of four normal female speakers reported in Fourakis (1991) for the same vowels produced bearing main stress and at slow tempo. As can be seen, RB's vowel formants correspond quite well with those of the normal female speakers. Thus, RB was able to produce vowels with appropriate formant structure, which certainly contributed to her high intelligibility scores. Figures 8 and 9 show RB's formant measurements taken at 10 equally spaced intervals, starting at the vowel onset, for two tokens each of the vowels [i] and [æ] in the [b_d] context. Her overall formant trajectories can be seen as the lines connecting the individual formant values. These plots are representative of the three vowels [i, e, æ] that were recorded in the C_d context. Only [æ] showed significant formant transitions for all three initial consonants.

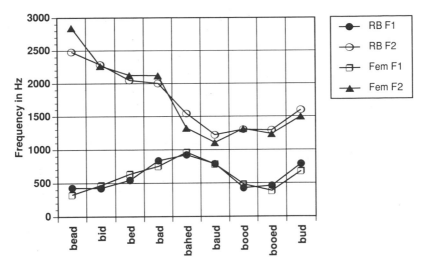

Figure 7. Mean frequencies of RB's first and second vowel formants as compared to those of four normal female speakers.

This vowel was the lowest, involving maximum excursion of the jaw. It can be seen in Figure 9 that the steady-state frequency of her second formant was achieved almost immediately, with a slight rise after 60 ms, while that of her first formant was achieved within 30 ms for the second repetition and within 70 ms for the first repetition. The situation was similar for the [g] context, while for the [d] context her first formant's steady-state fre-

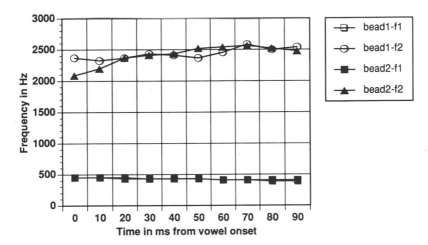

Figure 8. Formant measurements for RB taken at 10 equally spaced intervals, starting at vowel onset, for the vowel [i] in [b_d] context.

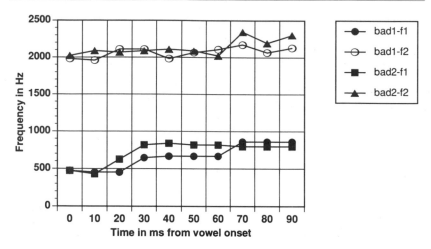

Figure 9. Formant measurements for RB taken at 10 equally spaced intervals, starting at vowel onset, for the vowel [æ] in [b_d] context.

quency was reached within 40 ms for both tokens. The range of 30–60 ms transition durations compares favorably with those reported by Kewley-Port (1982).

The carrier sentences were designed to elicit the test words in sentence-medial and sentence-final positions, in order to determine whether RB exhibited the phrase final lengthening that is typical in normal subjects (Wightman, Shattuck-Hufnagel, Ostendorf, & Price, 1992). Furthermore, the words "pap," "pab," "tap," "tab," "cap," and "cab" were included to see if she exhibited prevoiced consonant lengthening. Figure 10 shows the durations of initial closure, voice onset time, vowel, and final closure in sentence-medial and sentence-final position for all the C_d words, pooled across voicing and place of articulation of the initial consonant and across vowels. It can be seen that for all intervals, except the final closure, RB's medial segments were equal to or longer than her final segments. In addition, her closures for the initial consonants were extremely long. Thus, RB was not able to implement final lengthening. The timing results for the "pap," "pab" words showed that RB had longer vowels when the following consonant was [b] than when it was [p]. The mean vowel duration in words ending in voiced /b/ was 369 ms as opposed to 205 ms in words ending in voiceless /p/, regardless of position in the sentence, indicating that the phonological rule of vowel lengthening was applied, and its effects implemented. The results for the implementation of final lengthening were exactly the same as for the previously discussed set of words.

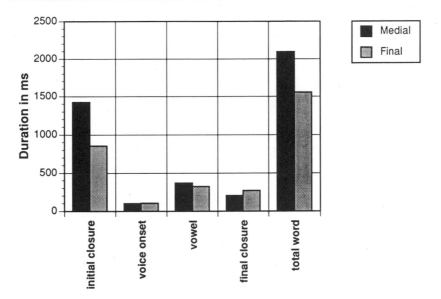

Figure 10. Durations of initial closure, voice onset time, vowel, and final closure in sentence medial and sentence final positions for all C_d words.

DISCUSSION

The results of this study demonstrate the clinical utility of combining different, but complementary, instrumental measures in the assessment of dysarthric speech. Based on the above findings the following observations are offered.

First, as stated earlier, the nature of closed head injuries typically results in a heterogeneous group of survivors with varied combinations of diffuse and focal brain injuries. With such patients instrumental assessment of multiple speech subsystems, as conducted in the present study, in conjunction with perceptual measures, may result in a more complete understanding of the pathophysiology of motor impairment and the concomitant dysarthria. This was certainly the case with RB. For example, the overall slowed rate of speech and nonspeech movements noted was consistent with involvement of the basal ganglia. Also, the decreased movement displacements and velocities for her upper and lower lips were consistent with her parkinsonian-like symptomatology. Thus, it seemed that some of the primary characteristics of her dysarthria, which could be objectively measured, may have been more attributable to her focal lesions than to diffuse damage.

Second, any supplementary instrumental measure should contribute diagnostically as well as toward treatment planning. The multiple measures employed in the present study did both. For example, measurement of movement frequency was consistent with, and confirmed objectively, RB's slowed rate of speech noted in the perceptual assessment. However, without these measures, the differential degree of impairment in movement displacement and velocity between lips and jaw could not have been detected and documented. Findings from the aerodynamic measures were inconsistent with the perceptual observation of reduced respiratory support for speech, and suggested another explanation for the phonatory symptoms of RB's dysarthria. Finally, the acoustic measures provided objective evidence for RB's relatively good intelligibility scores. Although more is better, in the interest of clinical practicality a limited number of carefully selected instrumental measures can yield a very comprehensive assessment of speech production.

Third, one of the advantages of studying a brain-injured individual who is several years postonset is that their impairments tend to be more chronic or stable in nature. When impairments are relatively stable, compensations, either volitional or not, are more easily identified. The subject studied in this investigation was 5 years post-onset of CHI. Over the course of assessment, decreased movement displacements of her upper and lower lips were noted, but were in marked contrast to displacements of her jaw, which were within the normal range. This discrepancy may have been the result of an adventitious process in which RB's speech mechanism attempted to compensate for her decreased lip closure by increasing jaw movement. The degree to which this mechanism improved her intelligibility was unclear. However, the nature of the measurements made lead to the identification of a clinical question and possible target for therapy. That is, could the intelligibility and/or the naturalness of RB's speech be improved by increasing lip strength? The authors will be exploring this question.

Finally, the question of whether or not an individual, who is five years post injury with single word and sentence intelligibility scores above 90%, might still be a candidate for remediation should be addressed. First, although intelligibility has been suggested as the best measure of disability in dysarthria (Yorkston et al., 1988), it may vary significantly when it is measured in natural settings (Berry & Sanders, 1983). Second, frequently individuals with dysarthria who have fair-to-good intelligibility scores also continue to demonstrate speaking patterns that are very distracting to the listener. This can have a significant psychological impact on the effectiveness of the communicative dyad. In the case of RB, both these factors were present. Her intelligibility tended to decrease outside the clinical setting and strangers had more difficulty with her speech than did her family. In addition, she was working part time as a benefits counselor for the Veterans' Administration and felt that her effectiveness was often diminished due to her speech. These issues, together with her willingness to continue therapy, and the potential remediation strategy identified by the instrumental measures, made RB a candidate for ongoing rehabilitative services.

REFERENCES

Baken, R. J. (1987). *Clinical measurement of speech and voice.* Boston: College-Hill.

Berry, W. R., & Saunders, S. B. (1983). Environmental education: The universal management approach for adults with dysarthria. In W. R. Berry (Ed.) *Clinical dysarthria* (pp. 203–216). San Diego: College-Hill.

Darley, F. L., Aronson, A. E., & Brown, J. R. (1975). *Motor speech disorders.* Philadelphia: W. B. Saunders.

Enderby, P. (1983). *Frenchay dysarthria assessment.* San Diego: College-Hill.

Fourakis, M. (1991). Tempo, stress, and vowel reduction in American English. *Journal of the Acoustical Society of America, 90,* 1816–1827.

Gerratt, B. R., Till, J. A., Rosenbek, J. C., Wertz, R. T., & Boysen, A. E. (1991). Use and perceived value of perceptual and instrumental measures in dysarthria management. In C. A. Moore, K. M. Yorkston, & D. R. Beukelman (Eds.), *Dysarthria and apraxia of speech: Perspectives on management* (pp. 77–93). Baltimore: Paul H. Brookes Publishing Co.

Keller, E. (1990). *Signalyze.* Seattle: InfoSignal, Inc.

Kewley-Port, D. (1982). Measurement of formant transitions in naturally produced stop consonant-vowel syllables. *Journal of the Acoustical Society of America, 72,* 379–389.

McNeil, M. R. (1986, February). *A critical appraisal of instrumentation methods in the evaluation and management of dysartyhria.* Paper presented at the Clinical Dysarthria Conference, Tucson, AZ.

Netsell, R., Lotz, W. K., & Barlow, S. M. (1989). A speech physiology examination for individuals with dysarthria. In K. M. Yorkston & D. R. Beukelman (Eds.), *Recent advances in clinical dysarthria.* Boston: College-Hill Press.

Wightman, C. W., Shattuck-Hufnagel, S., Ostendorf, M., & Price, P. J. (1992). Segmental durations in the vicinity of prosodic phrase boundaries. *Journal of the Acoustical Society of America, 91,* 1718–1726.

Yorkston, K. M., & Beukelman, D. R. (1981). *Assessment of intelligibility of dysarthric speech.* Tigard, OR: CC Publications.

Yorkston, K. M., Beukelman, D. R., & Bell, K. R (1988). *Clinical management of dysarthric speakers.* San Diego: College-Hill.

Chapter 9

Accelerometric Difference Index for Subjects with Normal and Hypernasal Speech

James A. Till, Mehdi Jafari, and Cindy B. Law-Till

THE TERM "HYPERNASALITY" implies abnormally large amounts of perceived nasal resonance in speech. Most commonly, patients with hypernasal speech have velopharyngeal insufficiency (VPI) because of congenital anomalies affecting the palate, surgical alterations of the velopharynx, or neurogenic disorders affecting the function of the velopharyngeal port. Clinical management of individuals with VPI is complex and often accomplished by a team of specialists including surgeons, prosthodontists, and speech pathologists (McWilliams, Morris, & Shelton, 1984).

Initial diagnostic evaluation of VPI requires assessment of velopharyngeal (VP) structure, VP physiologic function, and the speech abnormality. Endoscopic and radiographic techniques can provide information about velopharyngeal structure (Baken, 1987; McWilliams et al., 1984). Aerodynamic measures allow inferences about VP function during specific speech maneuvers. VP port area and resistance can be estimated by obtaining measures of oral pressures and nasal airflows during stop

This work was supported in part by the Rehabilitation Research and Development Service, Project C468-R, Department of Veterans Affairs, Washington, D.C. This chapter is in the public domain.

We thank Linda Alp, Arnold Yuan, and Paulette Metzger for their assistance in data collection and Lauren Truesdell for programming assistance.

consonant closure (Netsell, Lotz, & Barlow, 1989; Warren & DuBois, 1964).

Although each of the above techniques provides valuable information, none of them quantifies directly the severity of the functional deficit in speech. The severity of the speech deficit is important to measure both for planning management and monitoring the effects of treatment.

> An objective measure such as the one derived from the nasal accelerometer is probably a more reliable indication of the adequacy of velopharyngeal adjustment than a listener's judgment of this attribute. (Stevens, Kalikow, & Willemain, 1975, p. 411)

The concept of hypernasality is fundamentally perceptual in nature (Moll, 1964). However, in clinical practice, perceptual judgments from a single clinician may not quantify reliably the degree of hypernasality present (Bradford, Brooks, & Shelton, 1964; Colton & Cooker, 1968; Sherman, 1954). Measures that are known to correlate with group listener judgments of hypernasality must be established.

Attempts have been made to extract measures correlating with hypernasality from the speech spectrum. However, these attempts generally have been unsuccessful because variation in the nonvelar vocal tract configuration markedly affects the speech spectrum (Curtis, 1970). Other researchers have attempted to quantify hypernasality by measuring sound pressure levels (SPLs) emitted from the nose (Fletcher, 1970). In order to compensate for fluctuations in speech SPL, ratios or differences between nasal-oral SPL have been proposed. Shelton, Knox, Arndt, and Elbert (1967) found relatively low ($r < .50$) correlations between nasal-oral energy ratios and listener judgments. There are reports that filtered nasal-oral energy ratios show higher correlations (e.g., Dalston & Warren, 1986). However, as recently as 1987, Baken (p. 404) concluded that specific advantages of filtering nasal-oral energy ratios have not been demonstrated clearly.

Stevens et al. (1975) and Stevens, Nickerson, Boothroyd, and Rollins (1976) proposed using a miniature accelerometer taped to the subject's nose to obtain measures correlated with perceived hypernasality. In the 1976 study, 41 normal speaking children and adults demonstrated an average of 11–20 dB difference between peak accelerometer output on vowels compared to an /m/ reference token. In 12 samples of hearing-impaired childrens' speech known to have hypernasal quality, accelerometric measures and perceptual ratings of the hypernasal speech samples were correlated (Pearson $r = .78$). Lippmann (1981) also showed a mean accelerometric difference of about 15 dB between /m/ and vowels in normal speakers. Horii's initial work (1980, 1983) sought to compensate for the effects of vocal intensity by utilizing two channels of accelerometric signal; one on the throat, which transduced neck vibration during voiced signals, and one on the nose. He used a ratio of nasal-to-oral accelerometric amplitude scaled so that the prolonged /m/ for any given subject would yield a value of 1.0. This became known as the HONC index. The procedure addressed three of the main problems in accelerometry: 1) variation in tissue attenuation/transmission among patients, 2) variations in day-to-day placement and changes in accelerometric amplitude thereby induced, and 3) sensitivity to vocal amplitude. Horii (1983) obtained a correlation of 0.92 between perceptual scaling and the HONC measure in speakers simulating hypernasality. Redenbaugh and Reich (1985) and Reich (1985) utilized a similar measure, the Nasal Accelerometric Vibrational Index (NAVI), to obtain correlations of 0.85 and 0.90 with perceptual scaling of hypernasality. Moon (1990) has reported the effects of nasal airway patency on accelerometric data. Horii (1990) has stated that he believes dual transducer ratio methods may not be necessary if careful selection of stimulus materials and tasks are used to control for loudness variations.

Despite findings supporting the clinical utility of accelerometry to measure hypernasality, widespread application of the technique in the management of individuals with VPI has not occurred. This may be because initial reports utilized dual accelerometer channels and large laboratory computers to process the signals and derive the measures. Currently, there is no popular commercial device for accelerometric measurement. With increasing availability of personal computers in clinical environments, accelerometry can become more accessible to the clinician and patients with VPI. But, no protocol has been agreed upon. Ideally, accelerometric measurement should quantify the degree of hypernasality and classify different levels of hypernasality in a reliable fashion.

This chapter reports an accelerometric procedure utilizing one accelerometer, a simple task, and PC automated computer processing. Two experiments are reported. In experiment I the effects of speaking tasks and accelerometer placement/replacement were studied. Experiment II was based on the findings of experiment I and investigated the relationship between a new measure, the Accelerometer Difference Index (ADI), and direct magnitude estimation (DME) ratings of hypernasality.

EXPERIMENT I: SPEAKING TASKS
AND ACCELEROMETER PLACEMENT

The specific aims of this experiment were to: 1) compare nasal accelerometer amplitudes during various speaking tasks in normal and hypernasal speakers, and 2) investigate the effect of accelerometer placement/replacement.

Subjects

Five male American-English speakers with no history of speech, hearing, or neuromotor disorders (mean age = 29.8, SD = 7.5 years) and five male American-English speakers (mean age = 67.8, SD = 4.8 years) with hypernasal speech were studied. Previous research (Stevens et al., 1976) suggests that the rather large difference in mean age of the groups would not affect the accelerometric output. The subjects with hypernasal speech each had been evaluated by a certified speech-language pathologist who reported clinically significant hypernasality. No attempt was made to control for gender, age, etiology, or presence of other speech deviations. Each subject was sufficiently fluent to complete the Rainbow Passage (Fairbanks, 1960). On the basis of the available subjective clinical data, the subjects with hypernasal speech were selected to represent a range from mild to severe hypernasality. Table 1 documents the demographic and etiologic information for the subjects with hypernasal speech.

Procedure

Each subject was seated in a sound-treated booth (IAC Model 40). The speech and accelerometric signals were recorded on a Revox (Model B-77) tape recorder located outside the booth. The acoustic signal was sensed with a Revox M3500 microphone located 100 mm from the subject's mouth at approximately 45 degrees azimuth. Nasal vibrations were sensed with a miniature accelerometer (Knowles Electronics, BU-1771). This transducer weighs less than 1.8 g and has a −45 dB sensitivity (ref. 1.0 V/g) and a flat ±2.0 dB frequency response to 3000 Hz. The nasal accelerometer was taped firmly on the subject's left superior nares wall overlying the lateral nasal cartilage and immediately anterior to the nasal bone (Redenbaugh & Reich, 1985). This placement (position 6) has been found to be maximally sensitive to nasal vibration (Lippmann, 1981). The accelerometer output was preamplified by custom electronics and connected to one input channel of the tape recorder. The microphone was connected to the other channel. Tape recorder gain levels for both channels were constant throughout the experiment. The line level signals from the tape recorder were amplified (SA Instrumentation, Model SA-411) prior to

Table 1. Description of subjects with hypernasality

Name—code	Age (years)	Etiology	Time post-onset
SOG (H1)	64	Right CVA	5 years
RDS (H2)	65	Myopathy	25 years
SMM (H3)	64	Primary lateral sclerosis	6 years
AOJ (H4)	72	Left CVA	8 months
WLM (H5)	74	Brainstem CVA	12 years

digital sampling at 1 KHz with 12-bit quantization (RC Electronics, ISC-16). Analyses of the digitized signals were accomplished by custom software incorporated in the CASPER (Till, 1990) computer-assisted diagnostic assessment system.

Each subject completed: 1) the Rainbow Passage (Fairbanks, 1960); 2) three 32-second monologues; 3) five repetitions of a sentence loaded with nasal consonants, "No More Moms Near," (hereafter, "nasal sentence"); 4) five repetitions of a similar sentence with no nasal consonants, "Show Boats Bob Well," (hereafter, "non-nasal sentence"); 5) five repetitions of sustained /i/, /a/, and /u/; and 6) five isolated prolongations of /m/ for three seconds. After tasks 1–6 were completed, tasks 3, 4, 5, and 6 were repeated with replacement of the accelerometer. All the subjects were asked to perform the tasks at a relatively constant conversational effort level.

Data Analysis

The mean root mean square (rms) accelerometer voltage provided a unique reference signal, reflecting individual variations in transducer placement, tissue transmission, and damping characteristics. For each subject and task, the accelerometric data were expressed as a decibel pressure ratio with reference to the mean rms of the sustained productions of /m/. A separate reference voltage was obtained after transducer replacement.

Two separate algorithms for analysis of rms voltages were implemented for the monologue and the Rainbow Passage. The first calculated rms voltage for the entire sample, including both periods of silence and voiceless energy. The second analysis excluded periods of silence and voiceless energy, and computed mean rms values for 64-ms windows centered on each syllable nucleus. The sentence analyses were performed interactively using a microcomputer. The digitized records were displayed and manually segmented using the acoustic data. First, the beginning and end of the sentence were identified, then the voiceless segments were marked in order to exclude them from rms calculations. For the vowels and sustained /m/, the rms voltages were obtained from a 200-ms sample collected near the midpoint of the prolonged phonation.

Statistical comparisons between groups and among speaking tasks were accomplished with repeated measures analyses of variance (ANOVAs) and appropriate follow-up contrasts of individual means, if required. For all tests, an alpha level of .05 was used to infer statistical significance.

Results and Discussion: Experiment I

Table 2 shows the group means and standard deviations for each speaking condition during the initial transducer placement trial. Because the dB values were calculated relative to the /m/ reference voltage, negative dB

Table 2. Mean and standard deviation nasal accelerometer voltage ratio (dB re: /m/ calibration rms voltage) for each speaking task and group

| | Experimental task | | | | | | |
| | Monologue | | Rainbow | | Sentence | | |
	Total	Syllable	Total	Syllable	Non-nasal	Nasal	Vowels
Nondisabled							
M	−7.01	−10.08	−6.89	−9.68	−19.47	−4.28	−14.68
SD	2.75	2.83	3.12	3.12	2.87	1.47	2.26
Group with hypernasality							
M	−3.01	−3.84	−4.79	−3.75	−5.38	−3.51	−6.01
SD	2.81	2.24	3.49	2.38	5.28	3.07	2.67
Group difference							
	4.00	6.20*	2.10	5.93*	14.09*	0.77	8.67*

*Significant group difference (p <.05).

values of smaller magnitude imply increased nasal vibration. A group × task ANOVA revealed a significant main effect for group ($F = 21.95$, $df = 1,8$) and task ($F = 15.96$, $df = 6, 48$). Because there was a significant group × task interaction ($F = 8.64$, $df = 6, 48$), Cochran approximate t comparisons (Lindquist, 1956) of group means for each task were completed. Group differences (bottom of Table 2) that achieved statistical significance are marked with an asterisk. The results show that the syllable analysis improved separation of the groups for the monologue and Rainbow Passage tasks. However, the single-sentence task provided maximum group differentiation.

Data for accelerometer placement/replacement trials are shown in Table 3. There were no significant differences between trials for either group. Figure 1 shows the pattern of results obtained for the three vowels. The observed pattern is in conformity with other reported findings (Stev-

Table 3. Nasal accelerometer calibration voltage and voltage ratio (dB re calibration voltage) for the three experimental tasks repeated after initial placement (T1) and replacement (T2) of the accelerometer

| | Experimental task | | | | | | | |
| | Calibration volts | | Non-nasal sentence | | Nasal sentence | | Vowels | |
	T1	T2	T1	T2	T1	T2	T1	T2
Nondisabled								
M	2.10	2.12	−19.47	−18.99	−4.28	−3.95	−14.68	−13.20
SD	0.79	0.74	2.87	2.49	1.47	1.89	2.26	2.27
Group with hypernasality								
M	2.15	2.29	−5.38	−4.46	−3.51	−2.41	−6.01	−7.18
SD	0.60	0.61	5.28	6.09	3.07	3.48	2.67	4.35

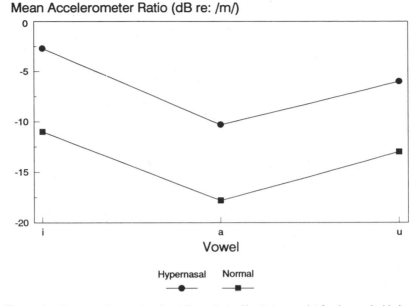

Mean Accelerometer Ratio (dB re: /m/)

Figure 1. Mean accelerometric values (dB re: /m/ calibration rms volts) for the nondisabled and hypernasal group during production of: 1) /i/; 2) /a/; and 3) /u/.

ens et al., 1976). They suggested that greater inherent nasal energy is present for vowels /i/ and /u/ because of their lower first formant frequency relative to the /a/ vowel. They also maintain that the acoustic impedance of the velopharyngeal port increases with frequency. Therefore, higher nasal energy and lower velopharyngeal acoustic impedance for /i/ and /u/ would result in larger accelerometer output relative to /a/.

EXPERIMENT II: ACCELEROMETRIC DIFFERENCE INDEX

The second experiment was designed to obtain DME ratings of hypernasality for the subjects with hypernasal speech and to test the correlation of an accelerometer measure to the DME ratings.

Accelerometric Difference Index

On the basis of Experiment I results, a new accelerometric measure, the ADI, was defined and tested. In Experiment I there was no significant difference in either group for nasal accelerometer voltage between the nasal sentence and the /m/ calibration conditions (see Table 2). This suggested that nasal sentence data could serve as individual calibration references for each subject. Therefore, the prolonged /m/ maneuver was eliminated. Because the sentence task resulted in the largest difference between groups in Experiment I, the two sentences were used to define ADI as follows:

$$ADI(dB) = 20 \times \log [(\text{rms accel. nasal sentence})/(\text{rms accel. non-} \quad (1)$$
$$\text{nasal sentence})]$$

The primary questions were: 1) Would ADI reliably separate normal from hypernasal speakers? and 2) To what extent would ADI values agree with DME perceptual judgments of hypernasality for speakers with disabilities?

Subjects

Data for the five speakers with hypernasality and five nondisabled speakers described in Experiment I were reanalyzed. IN addition, nine college students rated the speakers' hypernasality using DME. The judges were four males and five females (age: $M = 22.11$, $SD = 3.82$ years) without histories of speech or hearing disorders and with no experience listening to impaired speech. Each passed bilateral audiometric pure tone screening for 500, 1000, 2000, and 4000 Hz at 25 dB-HL (ANSI, 1970) in a sound-treated booth (IAC, model 1204A).

Procedures

DME Rating The DME rating was done in two steps: 1) determination of the anchor stimulus (medium hypernasality among patients) by professional judges, and 2) rating of the stimuli by naïve judges using the anchor stimulus as the reference. To determine the anchor stimulus, five certified speech pathologists independently ranked the patients with hypernasality for degree of hypernasality. One subject acquired the median rank by all the judges. Three sentences of a monologue by this subject were chosen as the anchor stimulus.

The first two sentences of the Rainbow Passage read by each subject were used for direct magnitude estimation of hypernasality. For each of the 10 speakers, five repetitions of the sentence pairs were dubbed from the original recording (Revox, Model BU-77) to a DME test tape (Marantz, model PMD-221). The order of the 50 sentence pairs was randomized. The anchor stimulus was interposed between each successive ten sentence-pairs.

The judges were tested individually in a sound-treated room (IAC Model 40). They were seated 1.5 m in front of a loud speaker (Yamaha, DM-01) at ear level. The judges were instructed to focus on hypernasality and disregard any consideration of abnormality in rate, clarity of pronunciation, intensity, pitch, or fluency. They were trained by listening to the anchor stimulus sentence representing moderate hypernasality with a pre-assigned scale value of 100, and by listening to four other samples of the same sentence. Two of the additional sentences had hypernasality levels greater than the anchor stimulus and two had hypernasality levels less than the anchor stimulus. They were free to listen to the training tape as many times as they needed until they felt comfortable completing the rating task. During the experimental rating task, the test stimuli were played consecutively, one at a time. The judges were allowed as much time as necessary to assign their rating. Each 10-sample block was followed by the anchor stimulus identified as such.

Because the nine judges were allowed to scale their DME ratings of perceived hypernasality independently, the raw DME data were normalized prior to analysis of the group data. The range used by each judge was constrained between 0 and 100 by dividing the raw DME scores from each judge by the maximum score assigned by him or her. Each subject's DME hypernasality score was acquired by averaging the ratings over each judge and then pooling over all judges.

Accelerometric Procedure The first three tokens for task 3, the nasal sentence, and task 4, the non-nasal sentence, were reanalyzed from the original tape records for acoustic and accelerometric signals. As in the previous experiment, the CASPER system (Till, 1990) was used for data acquisition and analysis. This system automatically detected sentence onset and offset and excluded nonvoiced portions. Then, mean windowed rms voltage was calculated for the voiced segments of the sentences. The mean ADI measure, as described above, was computed for each subject. As in Experiment I, statistical comparisons between groups were accomplished with repeated-measure ANOVAs and follow-up contrasts of individual means of alpha levels of $p = .05$.

RESULTS: EXPERIMENT II

ADI Results

The ADI means and standard deviations for each of the subjects with hypernasality and the nondisabled subjects are shown in Table 4. Group means and *SD*s are also shown. The ANOVA comparing group means was significant ($F = 17.40$, $df = 1, 8$). The ADI scatter plot shown in Figure 2 revealed no overlap between groups.

DME Results

Table 5 shows the mean normalized DME rating and standard deviation among judges for each speaker. Group means and *SD*s are also shown. ANOVA comparison of the group means revealed a significant group difference ($F = 24.07$, $df = 91, 8$). Figure 3 is the scatter plot of the DME

Mean Accelerometric Difference Index (ADI)

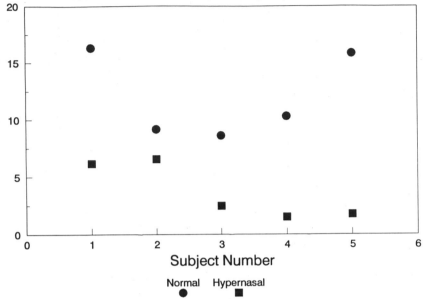

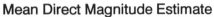

Figure 2. Scatter plot of ADI values for all subjects.

Mean Direct Magnitude Estimate

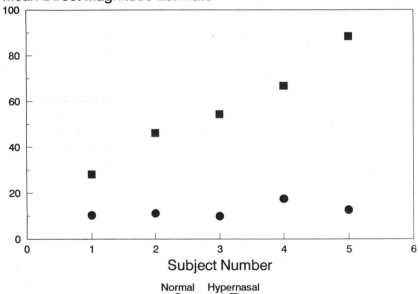

Figure 3. Scatter plot of mean normalized DME ratings for all subjects.

Correction for *Motor Speech Disorders: Advances in Assessment and Treatment*

The figure that appears on page 85 should appear as Figure 3 on page 86. The following figure should replace the one on page 85 as Figure 1.

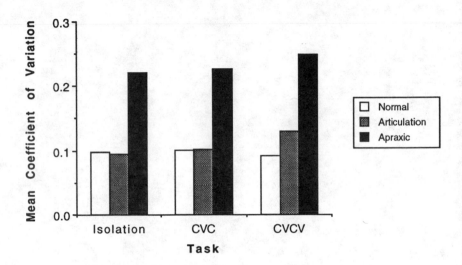

data. The perceptual comparisons also separated the groups studied with little overlap.

Relationship between ADI and DME Ratings

The results above show that both the ADI metric and the DME data from nine judges separated the nondisabled subjects from the subjects with hypernasality with no overlap. However, the analyses do not address the extent to which ADI quantifies the severity of perceived hypernasality. As a group, the professional judges ranked the subjects with hypernasality from H1 to H5 in order of increasing severity. Comparison of the ADI means (Table 4) and the DME ratings (Table 5) shows similar ranking in sequential order of severity for the hypernasal subjects. The one exception was a reversal in rank order for subjects H1 and H2. The small difference in mean ADI for these two subjects (0.38 dB) with respect to their *SD*s (2.11 for H1 and 2.26 for H2) suggests that their ADI rankings could be interpreted as essentially the same. Although limited by the few subjects, the ADI data in Table 4 suggest that the group with hypernasality may have represented at least three degrees of severity: 1) mild (H1, H2), 2) moderate (H3), and 3) severe (H4, H5). The DME results do not allow such clear classification. However, the perceived hypernasality increased systematically for subjects H1 through H5. Moreover, subject H3 was

Table 4. Mean and *SD* accelerometric difference index (ADI) for subjects with hypernasality and nondisabled subjects

Subject	ADI	
	Mean	SD
N1	16.32	4.20
N2	9.17	1.34
N3	8.61	3.26
N4	10.30	1.80
N5	15.83	1.60
Nondisabled group	12.05	3.73
H1	6.18	2.11
H2	6.56	2.26
H3	2.47	1.72
H4	1.50	0.45
H5	1.74	0.64
Group with hypernasality	3.69	2.48

Table 5. Mean normalized DME ratings and standard deviation among judges for each speaker

Subject	Normalized DME rating Mean	SD
N1	10.33	4.19
N2	11.15	4.05
N3	9.88	2.90
N4	17.43	5.46
N5	12.68	5.21
Nondisabled group	12.29	3.06
H1	28.16	4.31
H2	46.16	9.28
H3	54.36	6.47
H4	66.77	7.15
H5	88.35	10.44
Group with hypernasality	56.76	22.56

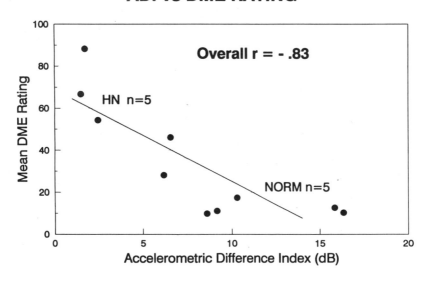

ADI vs DME RATING

Figure 4. Relationship of mean DME ratings to mean ADI values for speakers with hypernasality.

assigned median hypernasality by the professional judges, the naïve judges, and ADI.

Figure 4 shows the bivariate relationship of DME to ADI for the five subjects with hypernasality. The observed Pearson correlation coefficient of −0.82 is of the same magnitude reported by other researchers (Horii, 1983; Redenbaugh & Reich, 1985; Stevens et al., 1976). However, the small sample precludes strong interpretation of the correlation.

CONCLUSION

The results of this study regarding the possibility of supplementing traditional perceptual judgments of hypernasality with more objective instrumental measures are encouraging. In order to be of value, instrumental measures of hypernasality should separate speakers with hypernasality from nondisabled speakers and quantify the severity of hypernasality to some extent.

In the present study, the ADI measure resulted in a significant difference between the nondisabled speakers and those with hypernasality. More relevant to clinical application, there was no overlap in ADI values between the groups. Although the current results are based on only five subjects in each group, it seems that, for the tasks studied, ADI values less than seven indicate the presence of clinically significant hypernasality.

Testing the ability of instrumental measures to quantify the severity of hypernasality demands the use of human judges. Unfortunately, as discussed previously, many factors influence human judgment. In the present study, we provided training and rating instructions in an attempt to limit the influence of factors other than hypernasality. The mean DME rating observed for the anchor subject (H3) was 54.36, which compares favorably with his expected rating (50.00). This suggests that the DME training was effective. The judges, as a group, were able to separate the nondisabled speakers from the speakers with hypernasality using DME technique. In addition, the relative order of judged severity closely agreed with the rank ordering based on ADI. Although not tested statistically because of the small number of subjects, the ADI values for the group with hypernasality suggest three levels of severity. Finally, the correlation (−0.82) between the DME ratings and ADI values suggests that ADI may be a useful measure for quantification of hypernasality.

The initial reports of accelerometric assessment of hypernasality occurred more than 15 years ago. Despite findings suggestive of clinical utility, accelerometry has not been used substantially in clinical settings. Concerns have been raised about the idiosyncratic nature of each person's nasal structure and nasal tissue response to vocal tract energy. Concerns also have been stated regarding within-subject variability induced by accelerometer placement variations. The present results suggest that variability with placement and replacement of the accelerometer can be controlled. The ADI measure studied compares the accelerometric outputs for nasal and non-nasal tasks (i.e., calculates the logarithmic difference) and thus, in a way, it can be assumed that idiosyncratic effects would be rendered not significant. The nasal sentence used for reference in calculating ADI is probably more representative of usual speech performance than the comparatively less natural sustained /m/ maneuver. By using a nasal sentence as a reference, the elicitation procedure is simplified. If the nasal and non-nasal sentences are elicited sequentially in pairs, then potential drift in speech intensity would probably affect each sentence similarly. As suggested by Horii (1990), speech intensity effects can probably be controlled by instructions and task definition.

More than 25 years ago, Moll (1964) argued that hypernasality was fundamentally a perceptual construct. Curtis (1970) explained in detail why simple measures of the acoustic signal would not quantify hypernasality. We agree with both points. However, such reasoning does not automatically justify the sole use of human perceptual judgment to assess hypernasality. We agree with Stevens et al. (1976) that "[a]n objective measure such as the one derived from the nasal accelerometer is probably a more reliable indication of the adequacy of velopharyngeal adjustment than a listener's judgment of this attribute" (p. 411). Further investigations and more data are required to identify reliable, valid, and clinically feasible techniques for objective quantification of hypernasality.

REFERENCES

American National Standards Institute. (1970). *Specifications for audiometers* (ANSI S3.6-1969, R-1970). New York: Author.

Baken, R. J. (1987). *Clinical measurement of speech and voice*. San Diego: College-Hill.

Bradford, L. J., Brooks, A. R., & Shelton, R. L. (1964). Clinical judgment of hypernasality in cleft palate children. *Cleft Palate—Craniofacial Journal, 1*, 329–335.

Colton, R. H., & Cooker, H. S. (1968). Perceived nasality in the speech of the deaf. *Journal of Speech and Hearing Research, 11*, 553–559.

Curtis, J. F. (1970). Acoustics of nasalized speech. *Cleft Palate—Craniofacial Journal, 7*, 380–396.

Dalston, R. M., & Warren, D. W. (1986). Comparison of TONAR II, pressure-flow, and listener judgments of hypernasality in the assessment of velopharyngeal function. *Cleft Palate—Craniofacial Journal, 23*, 108–115.

Fairbanks, G. (1960). *Voice and articulation handbook*. New York: Harper & Row.

Fletcher, S. G. (1970). Theory and instrumentation for quantitative measurement of nasality. *Cleft Palate—Craniofacial Journal, 7*, 601–609.

Horii, Y. (1980). An accelerometric approach to nasality measurement: A preliminary report. *Cleft Palate—Craniofacial Journal, 17*, 254–261.

Horii, Y. (1983). An accelerometric measure as a physical correlate of perceived hypernasality in speech. *Journal of Speech and Hearing Research, 26,* 476–480.

Horii, Y. (1990). Commentary on accelerometry. *Cleft Palate—Craniofacial Journal, 27,* 270–274.

Lindquist, E. F. (1956). *Design and analysis of experiments in psychology and education.* Boston: Houghton Mifflin.

Lippmann, R. P. (1981). Detecting nasalization using a low-cost miniature accelerometer. *Journal of Speech and Hearing Research, 24,* 314–317.

McWilliams, B. J., Morris, H., & Shelton, R. (1984). *Cleft palate speech.* Philadelphia, PA: B. C. Decker.

Moll, K. L. (1964). "Objective" measures of nasality. *Cleft Palate—Craniofacial Journal, 1,* 371–374.

Moon, J. (1990). The influence of nasal patency on accelerometric transduction of nasal bone vibration. *Cleft Palate—Craniofacial Journal, 27,* 266–270.

Netsell, R., Lotz, W., & Barlow, S. (1989). A speech physiology examination for individuals with dysarthria. In K. M. Yorkston, & D. R. Beukelman (Eds.), *Recent advances in clinical dysarthria* (pp.3–37). Boston: College-Hill.

Redenbaugh, M., & Reich, A. R. (1985). Correspondence between an accelerometric nasal/voice amplitude ratio and listeners' direct magnitude estimations of hypernasality. *Journal of Speech and Hearing Research, 28,* 273–281.

Reich, A. R. (1985). Relation between accelerometric values and interval estimates of hypernasality. *Cleft Palate—Craniofacial Journal, 22,* 237–245.

Shelton, R. L., Knox, A. W., Arndt, W. B., & Elbert, M. (1967). The relationship between nasality score values and oral and nasal sound pressure level. *Journal of Speech and Hearing Research, 10,* 549–557.

Sherman, D. (1954). The merits of backward playing of connected speech in the scaling of voice quality disorders. *Journal of Speech and Hearing Disorders, 19,* 312–321.

Stevens, K. N., Kalikow, D. N., & Willemain, T. R. (1975). A miniature accelerometer for detecting glottal waveforms and nasalization. *Journal of Speech and Hearing Research, 18,* 594–599.

Stevens, K. N., Nickerson, R. S., Boothroyd, A., & Rollins, A. M. (1976). Assessment of nasalization in the speech of deaf children. *Journal of Speech and Hearing Research, 19,* 393–415.

Till, J. A. (1990). Computer-assisted evaluation of speech disorders: Rationale and directions for future development. *Journal for Computer Users in Speech and Hearing, 4,* 138–148.

Warren, D., & DuBois, A. (1964). A pressure-flow technique for measuring velopharyngeal orifice area during continuous speech. *Cleft Palate—Craniofacial Journal, 1,* 52–71.

Chapter 10

Increasing the Efficiency of Articulatory Force Testing of Adults with Traumatic Brain Injury

Monica A. McHenry,
John T. Minton, III, and Robin L. Wilson

TRAUMATIC BRAIN INJURY (TBI) often has devastating effects on the motor speech production system. The diffuse nature typical of the injury yields dysarthric patterns that do not conform to conventional categorization.

From a clinical perspective, particularly when working with an individual with TBI, efficient yet comprehensive testing is critical. The respiratory, laryngeal, velopharyngeal, and articulatory systems must be assessed individually to determine the pattern of deficits and to guide intervention. With the development of more sophisticated instrumentation (Barlow & Abbs, 1983), it is possible to objectify many aspects of the speech production system, rather than to rely solely upon observational or perceptual assessment. This new technology has provided a plethora of measures. Inherent redundancy among these measures has not been explored.

Objective testing of articulatory force is one of the more time-consuming portions of the comprehensive evaluation. An individual's ability to match and sustain four target force levels is assessed. In the force-

Supported by the Moody Foundation, Grant No. 91-15.

testing protocol, data are obtained at each of the following target force levels: 0.25 newton (N), 0.5 N, 1.0 N, and 2.0 N. These levels sample the range of articulatory forces typically generated during normal speech production (Barlow & Burton, 1990). Typically, 10 trials are obtained at each target force level (Barlow & Burton, 1990). Even when reduced to the minimum required for statistical significance (S.M. Barlow, personal communication, December 7, 1989), seven trials must be performed at each force level for each articulator. For normal subjects, assessment at each level for a given articulator could take as little as one minute, depending upon time between trials. For individuals with TBI, however, testing is often interrupted by breaks to increase or maintain arousal, to answer the individual's need to swallow, or to remove the bite block. Retesting of a trial is frequently required because of cognitive processing difficulties, impulsivity, and lack of attention or concentration during the task. Obtaining seven trials of valid data at a given force level can take as long as 15 minutes.

Eliminating separate testing of each articulator may not be an option to increase efficiency of an assessment protocol. It is well known clinically, especially for individuals who have sustained a TBI, that differential impairment exists among each of the physiological systems involved in speech production. It is of great clinical interest to know which system, or which structure within the articulatory system, evidences the greatest deficit. For example, if an individual's lower versus upper lip were more involved, one may expect a more severe intelligibility problem due to the lower lip's more active role in speech production. However, because it is relatively easy to compensate for labial deficits physiologically, greater impairment of the tongue may present a more challenging intervention problem.

A streamlined testing protocol must also continue to provide useful information regardless of severity of the subject's deficit. It is possible that performance on tasks at different force levels may vary according to severity of the subject's TBI. For example, more intelligible subjects may evidence poor contractile stability at only the 2.0 N level. If this were the case, elimination of the 2.0 N force level would lead to an incomplete articulatory force profile for more intelligible subjects.

With these considerations in mind, the present study was designed to determine if routinely obtained articulatory force measures could be grouped. The following questions were posed. First, is there a significant difference in force measures among the four testing levels of the protocol? Second, is the difference comparable between more and less intelligible groups of subjects with TBI?

METHODS

Subjects

The subjects were 17 males and 8 females who sustained severe TBI and who were consecutively admitted to a residential rehabilitation program. The only criteria for inclusion in the investigation were that the subject had suffered a traumatic brain injury and could complete the testing protocol. Subject characteristics are found in Table 1.

Table 1. Subject characteristics

Subject number	Sex	Age (years)	Months post-injury	Intelligibility (%)
1	F	33	36	96
2	M	35	30	93
3	M	22	13	90
4	F	27	6	84
5	M	21	4	82
6	F	20	84	78
7	M	23	14	74
8	F	21	30	73
9	M	29	120	72
10	M	21	36	72
11	M	19	7	70
12	M	20	4	59
13	F	22	24	58
14	M	20	30	56
15	F	22	66	55
16	M	22	30	54
17	M	19	72	52
18	F	22	42	43
19	M	20	42	39
20	M	25	13	34
21	M	34	108	30
22	M	18	12	28
23	M	27	60	22
24	F	27	228	19
25	M	18	6	6
Group x̄		23.5	44.7	57.5
SD		4.9	49.8	24.8
Male (n=17)	x̄	23.1	35.4	54.9
SD		5.2	35.5	25.2
Female (n=8)	x̄	24.3	64.5	63.1
SD		4.4	70.4	24.8

Subjects were grouped according to their scores on the Computerized Assessment of Intelligibility of Dysarthric Speech (CAIDS) (Yorkston, Beukelman, & Traynor, 1984) single-word test. Responses were judged by two naïve listeners with neither formal training in speech nor experience in communicating with individuals with dysarthria. Interjudge agreement, determined by comparing the two judges' intelligibility scores for three subjects, was 94%. Intrajudge reliability, determined by rejudging 25 utterances each of a less intelligible and a more intelligible subject, was 86% and 87%, respectively.

As seen in Table 1, a natural break in intelligibility scores is evident around 60%. Fourteen subjects with scores below 60% were placed in Group 1, the less intelligible group. Eleven subjects with scores above 60% were placed in Group 2, the more intelligible group.

Testing Protocol

Upon admission to the facility, each individual underwent a comprehensive motor speech evaluation. Assessment consisted of laryngeal and velopharyngeal resistance estimation, ramp and hold articulatory force testing, and audiotaping of the CAIDS single-word and sentence intelligibility test.

Instrumentation

The ramp and hold articulatory force testing is the focus of the present investigation. The transduction systems used to measure articulatory force have been described previously (Barlow & Rath, 1985). For upper and lower lip force measurement, a load-sensitive cantilever is attached to a yoke the subject holds between the teeth to minimize jaw contribution to the measure. Barlow and Netsell (1986) have illustrated the upper and lower lip transduction systems. For tongue force measurement, the jaw is again stabilized, with the tongue pushing anteriorly and superiorly against the cantilever. The tongue force transduction system is illustrated in Figure 1.

An 80386 microcomputer-based data acquisition and stimulus control system (Barlow, Suing, Grossman, Bodmer, & Colbert, 1989) was used to acquire force data. The analog force data were digitized on-line at 200 samples/sec after 50 Hz low pass filtering. Additional technical details of the data acquisition and analysis systems may be found elsewhere (Barlow & Burton, 1990; Barlow & Netsell, 1986; Barlow & Suing, 1991).

Data Acquisition

Target force levels delivered to an oscilloscope were presented to the subjects on a 19-inch black and white television. The subjects were in-

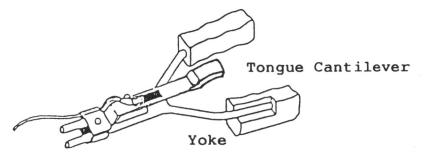

Figure 1. Tongue force transduction system.

structed to match the visual target as quickly and as accurately as possible by pushing against the cantilever. A schematic of the data acquisition system is provided in Figure 2. In the force-testing protocol, seven trials were obtained for the upper lip, lower lip, and tongue at each of the following target force levels: 0.25 N, 0.5 N, 1.0 N, and 2.0 N. (Jaw data were also obtained, but not reported in this study.)

In a typical trial, subjects evidenced some lag between the onset of the target and the onset of force generation. The ramp phase consisted of subjects increasing force quickly, usually overshooting the target. In the subsequent hold phase, subjects attempted to maintain the target force as

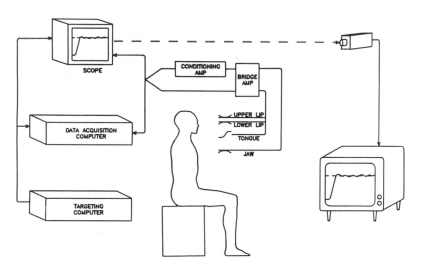

Figure 2. Data acquisition system.

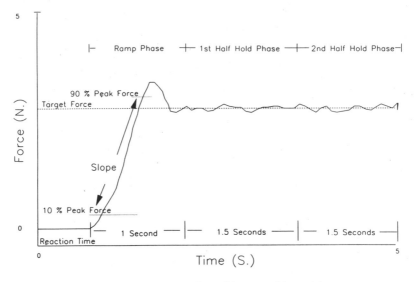

Figure 3. Measures obtained from typical force trial.

steadily as possible. Trial duration was five seconds. An example of a force trial with measures illustrated is presented in Figure 3. Each measure was averaged across the seven trials. Physiologic measures quantified from the digitized force records are defined in Table 2.

Statistical Analysis

Means and standard deviations of the seven trials were obtained for each force measure of interest. These data are presented in Table 3. For statistical analysis, subjects were grouped according to intelligibility regardless of gender. According to Barlow and Burton's (1990) study of 20 males and 20

Table 2. Physiologic measures and definitions

Reaction Time—time between the appearance of the target and the onset of articulatory movement

Slope—average rate of force change between 10% and 90% of peak force for a single trial

Derivative—fastest rate of force change between 10% and 90% of peak force for a single trial

Overshoot—peak force generated during the ramp phase

First Half Hold—average force during a 1.5 second interval beginning 1 second after the onset of articulatory movement

Second Half Hold—average force during a 1.5 second interval beginning 2.5 seconds after the onset of articulatory movement

First Half Standard Deviation (SD)—average variability during the first half-hold phase

Second Half SD—average variability during the second half-hold phase

Table 3. Data for physiologic measures

		Reaction time		Slope		Derivative		Overshoot	
		Group 1[a]	Group 2[b]	Group 1	Group 2	Group 1	Group 2	Group 1	Group 2
0.25 N	X̄	0.70	0.86	1.00	1.27	2.56	3.00	0.40	0.36
	SD	0.34	0.33	0.84	1.43	1.60	2.62	0.20	0.21
0.50 N	X̄	0.59	0.72	1.40	1.51	3.73	3.96	0.65	0.59
	SD	0.24	0.27	0.98	1.25	1.87	2.74	0.15	0.25
1.0 N	X̄	0.50	0.67	2.42	2.39	5.87	7.16	1.17	1.06
	SD	0.15	0.25	1.46	2.00	1.96	5.66	0.18	0.36
2.0 N	X̄	0.53	0.65	4.31	3.93	12.06	11.44	2.09	1.78
	SD	0.15	0.25	2.15	3.21	4.85	7.01	0.40	0.58
		1st 1/2 M		2nd 1/2 M		1st 1/2 SD		2nd 1/2 SD	
0.25 N	X̄	0.27	0.18	0.26	0.17	0.04	0.04	0.03	0.04
	SD	0.12	0.06	0.12	0.06	0.02	0.04	0.02	0.03
0.50 N	X̄	0.51	0.39	0.51	0.39	0.06	0.07	0.04	0.05
	SD	0.11	0.08	0.11	0.08	0.04	0.05	0.03	0.04
1.0 N	X̄	0.99	0.80	0.98	0.82	0.09	0.12	0.08	0.11
	SD	0.12	0.18	0.11	0.16	0.05	0.06	0.05	0.07
2.0 N	X̄	1.84	1.53	1.89	1.62	0.20	0.25	0.19	0.23
	SD	0.25	0.48	0.25	0.44	0.11	0.12	0.11	0.15

[a] Group 1—More intelligible subjects.
[b] Group 2—Less intelligible subjects.

141

females, gender differences occurred only at the maximum effort force level, a finding not addressed in this investigation.

Two-way (intelligibility group × force level) analyses of variance (ANOVAs) with repeated measures on one factor (force level) were performed for each measure. The Scheffé, a test "which sets the experimentwise error rate at α against all possible linear contrasts, not just pair-wise contrasts" (Howell, 1982, p. 303), was used for post-hoc testing. Simple effect calculations were completed to interpret the interaction effects (Howell, 1982). Partial correlation coefficients (SAS, 1988) were used to determine the relationship among the four target force levels.

RESULTS

Table 4 reports ANOVA results. A p value of .01 was employed to interpret all significance testing. Group main effects and group × force interactions are discussed for each measure. The results are presented chronologically across the ramp and hold phases. The force level main effect was significant for all measures. These results, as well as the correlation analyses among force levels, are discussed separately.

Reaction time is the time between the appearance of the target and the onset of articulatory movement. Group 1, the less intelligible group, evidenced significantly slower reaction time than Group 2, the more intelligible group. There was no group × force interaction.

Two related measures typically obtained during the ramp phase of articulatory movement are slope and first derivative. Slope indicates the average rate of force change during the ramp phase of a trial. The peak of the first derivative function indicates the fastest rate of force change. There were no group differences in these measures, nor was the group × force interaction significant. Continuing in chronologic order within the ramp and hold force task is overshoot, or the maximum force generated during a trial. The group main effect was significant, with the more intel-

Table 4. F ratios and p values for physiologic measures

	Force level main effect		Group main effect		Force × group interaction	
	F	p	F	p	F	p
Reaction time	23.13	.0001	7.00	.0102	0.34	.7197
Slope	75.10	.0001	0.00	.9796	0.82	.4348
Derivative	140.57	.0001	0.18	.6767	1.35	.2629
Overshoot	660.52	.0001	3.92	.0522	5.18	.0112
1st 1/2 M	885.95	.0001	22.56	.0001	4.83	.0262
2nd 1/2 M	1141.31	.0001	20.29	.0001	3.95	.0448
1st 1/2 SD	134.08	.0001	3.81	.0553	1.96	.1560
2nd 1/2 SD/M	101.35	.0001	3.28	.0747	1.32	.2644

ligible subjects evidencing higher values than the less intelligible individuals. Analysis of the group × force interaction revealed that the less intelligible subjects tended to undershoot the target, particularly at the 2.0 N level.

In the hold phase of the testing paradigm, the subject is to hold the target force as steadily as possible. First-half mean hold assesses the subject's ability to maintain the target force in the initial phase of the hold task. Fatigue effects may be evident in the second-half mean hold phase. Group main effects were significant for both the first- and second-half phases, with the less intelligible individuals sustaining lower target forces than the more intelligible subjects. The group × force level interaction reached significance for both phases as well. An analysis of simple effects revealed that for the first- and second-half phases, subjects differed significantly on each level, with the greatest difference between groups at the 2.0 N level.

Standard deviation is an indicator of the stability with which the subject held the target force. The same significance pattern was evident for both the first- and second-half hold phases. The group main effect did not reach significance, nor was there a significant group × force interaction for either the first- or second-half hold phases. Again, group differences were apparent, with less intelligible subjects evidencing less stability than more intelligible subjects. The group × force interaction did not reach significance.

Because one goal of this investigation was to determine the inherent redundancy among the four force levels, partial correlation matrices were generated for each measure. The correlation coefficients were used to determine if one force level was significantly related to any other. For reaction time, slope, derivative, and overshoot, all force levels were significantly correlated with one another. A representative matrix (overshoot) is presented in Table 5. For measures of mean hold and standard deviation for the first- and second-half phases, the 2.0 N level was not signifi-

Table 5. Force level correlation matrix and significance levels for overshoot

	Overshoot			
df = 63	2.0 N	1.0 N	0.5 N	0.25 N
2.0 N	1.000000 0.0	0.760848 0.0001	0.620530 0.0001	0.540719 0.0001
1.0 N	0.760848 0.0001	1.000000 0.0	0.721312 0.0001	0.623308 0.0001
0.5 N	0.620530 0.0001	0.721312 0.0001	1.000000 0.0	0.724660 0.0001
0.25 N	0.540719 0.0001	0.623308 0.0001	0.724660 0.0001	1.000000 0.0

cantly correlated with the 0.25 N level. In the case of standard deviation for the second-half phase, neither was the 2.0 N level correlated with the 0.5 N level. Correlation matrices for these measures are presented in Tables 6 and 7.

DISCUSSION

This investigation was designed to determine if the efficiency of articulatory force testing could be improved. The first specific question related to the potential significant difference in force measures among the four testing levels of the protocol. This was addressed by correlating the force levels among one another. Results indicated that only the 2.0 N force level differed significantly from any other force level. Each of the lower three levels was significantly related to one another.

The second specific question addressed differential performance on force levels according to intelligibility. Significant group × force interactions were present for the first- and second-half mean hold phases, where less intelligible subjects sustained lower forces at the 2.0 N force level. Interaction effects were also evident for overshoot, with less intelligible subjects undershooting the 2.0 N force level target.

Based on the above results, it may be concluded that information provided by any one of the lower three force levels would be representative of the subject's performance on the other two lower force levels. Because the group × force interactions did not involve the lower three force levels, information distinguishing more or less intelligible subjects would not be lost by testing only one of the lower levels. The 2.0 N level, on the other hand, seems to be an important differentiator between more and less intelligible subjects.

It is therefore suggested that the articulatory testing protocol could be reduced to testing at the 0.5 N and 2.0 N force levels. The 0.5 level is proposed rather than the 0.25 level because it is easier to administer accurately. Subjects frequently have difficulty returning completely to baseline following force generation. The problem is particularly apparent at the 0.25 level because of the very small increment between the subject's baseline and target force.

It is important to bear in mind that these results are confined to adults with TBI. Given a more varied caseload or subject pool, the discriminatory nature of the force levels may vary. The essential number of force levels will depend upon the clinical or research questions.

A more important clinical issue may be the relationship between articulatory force control and intelligibility following TBI. Although group differences were apparent for several measures, they are not addressed in this chapter. There are more appropriate analyses to assess

Table 6. Force level correlation matrices and significance levels for first- and second-half mean hold

	First-half mean hold			
df = 63	2.0 N	1.0 N	0.5 N	0.25 N
2.0 N	1.000000 0.0	0.751638 0.0001	0.357191 0.0035	0.258972 0.0372
1.0 N	0.751638 0.0001	1.000000 0.0	0.730399 0.0001	0.536837 0.0001
0.5 N	0.357191 0.0035	0.730399 0.0001	1.000000 0.0	0.809450 0.0001
0.25 N	0.258972 0.0372	0.536837 0.0001	0.809450 0.0001	1.000000 0.0
	Second-half mean hold			
df = 63	2.0 N	1.0 N	0.5 N	0.25 N
2.0 N	1.000000 0.0	0.716869 0.0001	0.500765 0.0001	0.288260 0.0199
1.0 N	0.716869 0.0001	1.000000 0.0	0.811449 0.0001	0.579935 0.0001
0.5 N	0.500765 0.0001	0.811449 0.0001	1.000000 0.0	0.841134 0.0001
0.25 N	0.288260 0.0199	0.579935 0.0001	0.841134 0.0001	1.000000 0.0

Table 7. Force level correlation matrices and significance levels for first- and second-half standard deviation

	First-half SD			
df = 63	2.0 N	1.0 N	0.5 N	0.25 N
2.0 N	1.000000 0.0	0.526819 0.0001	0.403128 0.0009	0.285330 0.0212
1.0 N	0.526819 0.0001	1.000000 0.0	0.575055 0.0001	0.410500 0.0007
0.5 N	0.403128 0.0009	0.575055 0.0001	1.000000 0.0	0.597055 0.0001
0.25 N	0.285330 0.0212	0.410500 0.0007	0.597055 0.0001	1.000000 0.0
	Second-half SD			
df = 63	2.0 N	1.0 N	0.5 N	0.25 N
2.0 N	1.000000 0.0	0.495832 0.0001	0.238366 0.0559	0.182438 0.1458
1.0 N	0.495832 0.0001	1.000000 0.0	0.710358 0.0001	0.585762 0.0001
0.5 N	0.238366 0.0559	0.710358 0.0001	1.000000 0.0	0.667966 0.0001
0.25 N	0.182438 0.1458	0.585762 0.0001	0.667966 0.0001	1.000000 0.0

differences between more and less intelligible subjects. For example, it is of interest to know if the articulatory force of more and less intelligible subjects differs according to articulatory structure as well as by force level. It will also be valuable to correlate the force measures with intelligibility to determine if certain measures predict grouping. We are currently assessing the relationships among articulatory strength, control, and intelligibility. The results of these investigations will contribute to more efficient assessment and intervention strategies for individuals with motor speech deficits.

REFERENCES

Barlow, S.M., & Abbs, J.H. (1983). Force transducers for the evaluation of labial, lingual, and mandibular motor impairments. *Journal of Speech and Hearing Research, 26,* 616–621.

Barlow, S.M., & Burton, M.K. (1990). Ramp-and-hold force control in the upper and lower lips: Developing new neuromotor assessment applications in traumatically brain injured adults. *Journal of Speech and Hearing Research, 33,* 660–675.

Barlow, S.M., & Netsell, R.L. (1986). Differential fine force control of the upper and lower lips. *Journal of Speech and Hearing Research, 29,* 163–169.

Barlow, S.M., & Rath, E. (1985). Maximum voluntary closing forces in the upper and lower lips of humans. *Journal of Speech and Hearing Research, 28,* 373–376.

Barlow, S.M., & Suing, G. (1991). FORCE: Automated digital signal processing program for parametric analysis of muscle forces in the orofacial mechanism. *Journal for Computer Users in Speech and Hearing, 7,* 228–250.

Barlow, S.M., Suing, G., Grossman, A., Bodmer, P., & Colbert, R. (1989). A high-speed data acquisition and protocol control system for vocal tract physiology. *Journal of Voice, 3,* 283–293.

Howell, D.C. (1982). *Statistical methods for psychology.* Boston: Duxbury Press.

SAS Institute Inc. (1988). *SAS/STAT User's guide, release 6.03 edition* [Computer program]. Cary, NC: SAS Institute Inc.

Yorkston, K.M., Beukelman, D.R., & Traynor, C.D. (1984). *Computerized assessment of intelligibility of dysarthric speech.* Austin, TX: PRO-ED.

Chapter 11

Tongue Function Testing in Parkinson's Disease
Indications of Fatigue

Nancy Pearl Solomon,
Donald A. Robin, Daryl M. Lorell,
Robert L. Rodnitzky, and Erich S. Luschei

THE ROLE OF weakness and fatigue in motor speech disorders is relatively unexplored. We have developed three techniques to evaluate the tongue for strength, endurance, and effort. This chapter is part of a larger project examining these functions in relation to speech and its disorders. The clinical relevance of these measures is being evaluated as well. The first two techniques, measures of strength and endurance, have been the focus of much of our work. The third measure, pertaining to the perception of effort, is new to our test battery.

All three techniques use the Iowa Oral Performance Instrument (IOPI, available through Breakthrough, Inc., 131 Technology Innovation Center, Oakdale, Iowa 52319) to obtain measures of pressure exerted by the tongue and the hand. The IOPI is a pressure-sensing instrument with a digital display (in kPa) and an LED display. Detailed descriptions of the IOPI can be found in Robin, Somodi, and Luschei (1991) and Robin, Goel, Somodi, and Luschei (1992). The tongue is tested because of its obvious relation to speech. The preferred hand is tested to ascertain if the findings can be generalized to other parts of the body.

This research was supported by Grant No. R03 DC01182 and Grant No. P60 DC00976 from the National Institutes on Deafness and Other Communication Disorders. We gratefully acknowledge the assistance of Lori B. Somodi, Samuel K. Seddoh, Daniel L. Keyser, and Judith K. Dobson.

147

For measures of maximum strength, subjects squeeze a small air-filled bulb as hard as they can. The tongue bulb is placed against the hard palate immediately posterior to the alveolar ridge and the subject pushes against the bulb with the anterior dorsum of the tongue. The hand bulb is placed in the palm of the preferred hand, and the subject wraps his or her fingers around the bulb and squeezes.

Endurance is assessed by measuring the subject's ability to maintain a pressure exertion on the bulb at 50% of his or her maximum strength. The IOPI is set up, by means of the digital display, so that the middle light on the LED display corresponds to 50% of the maximum pressure. The subject is instructed to squeeze the bulb so that the middle light is illuminated, and to keep it lit as long as possible. When the subject can no longer maintain 50% of maximum pressure, the trial is terminated. This measure should be a good indication of fatigue because, by definition, fatigue is a "failure to maintain the required or expected force" (Edwards, 1981).

Speech samples are recorded routinely as part of the tongue function evaluation. These involve syllable, word, phrase, and sentence repetitions for intelligibility analysis. In addition, a description of the "Cookie Theft" picture (Goodglass & Kaplan, 1981) is used for speech rate (calculated as the number of syllables produced per second excluding pauses >250 ms) and perceptual characteristics. Possible relationships between tongue function and speech impairment can be explored using this information.

To date, several studies from our laboratory have used a standardized protocol for the assessment of tongue and hand strength and endurance (Robin et al., 1991) in normal and disordered speakers. Lorell, Solomon, et al. (1992) and Solomon, Lorell, Robin, Rodnitzky, and Luschei (submitted) reported weaker than normal tongues but normal tongue endurance for a group of subjects with mild-to-moderate Parkinson's disease. Lorell and Robin (unpublished observations, July 1992) have documented reductions in tongue strength related to motor system degeneration in a patient with amyotrophic lateral sclerosis. Lorell, Robin, Somodi, Solomon, and Luschei (1992) observed reductions in tongue strength as a function of normal aging. Robin et al. (1991) found that children with developmental apraxia of speech had normal tongue strength, but significantly reduced endurance compared to normally speaking children. In contrast, Robin et al. (1992) documented increased endurance in subjects with exceptional skill with the tongue (debaters and trumpet players).

We have recently developed the third measure, an index of perceived effort, which we believe may have clinical utility. The evaluation of sense of effort was motivated by the obvious increase in effort that occurs during the endurance task. The fact that increased effort invariably accompanies tasks involving sustained muscular contractions with a constant force output has lead to revised definitions of fatigue that include both peripheral and central components. Enoka and Stuart (1985) define fatigue as "a progressive increase in the effort required to exert a desired force and the eventual progressive inability to maintain this force in sustained or repeated contractions" (p. 2281). Perception of effort is thought to be due to an awareness of descending motor drive by means of central feedback (e.g., Gandevia, 1982; McCloskey, 1981). If effort is high and prolonged, fatigue is experienced regardless of the state of muscle contraction. This is referred to as "central fatigue."

Reports of effort and fatigue in people with neurologic disease, in combination with the inability to sustain a task, may indicate a mismatch between descending motor commands and force production at the periphery. It has been suggested that performance of complex motor patterns relies on the programming of effort as an integral part of volitional output (McCloskey, 1981). Neilson and O'Dwyer (1984) hypothesized that abnormal internal feedback may play a part in the abnormal movements of individuals with athetoid cerebral palsy.

The task we have developed for assessing perceived effort involves squeezing the IOPI bulb to various levels of effort (from 10% to 90% of maximum in 10% increments). A visual display, in the guise of a thermometer, was used to cue subjects by marking the target effort level before each trial. Effort levels were tested in random order. A study using this technique was conducted with 20 young, healthy subjects (Somodi, Robin, & Luschei, submitted). Findings indicated a highly consistent sense of effort within and across subjects that related well to the actual pressures produced. The mathematical function describing the relation between effort and pressure was a third-order polynomial. Specifically, the function was continuously rising with a relatively flat midsection. This suggests that the low and high extremes of effort are more sensitive for pressure changes than is the range from approximately 30% to 80% of maximum effort. Of interest was that knowledge of 100% effort was not needed to calibrate submaximal effort levels. Similar results were obtained for both the tongue and the hand.

People with Parkinson's disease often report feelings of fatigue and increased effort while performing daily life activities (Mayeux et al., 1986; McDowell, 1971). Weakness, fatigue, and perceptions of effort in the use of the tongue may relate to some speech characteristics of hypokinetic dysarthria, especially imprecision of articulation (Canter, 1965; Darley, Aronson, & Brown, 1975; Logemann, Fisher, Boshes, & Blonsky, 1978; Solomon & Hixon, 1993). In our study of 23 people with mild-to-moderate Parkinson's disease (Lorell, Solomon, et al., 1992), we were surprised to find no difference between subjects with Parkinson's disease and control subjects for tongue and hand endurance. To explore the basis for the perceptions of fatigue further, we conducted follow-up studies with three of the subjects who reported fatigue. Subjects were tested again for strength and endurance and a speech sample was collected. In addition, the subjects performed the task for perceived effort.

In this preliminary report, we present the cases of three subjects with mild parkinsonism and complaints of fatigue, and data from three neurologically normal control subjects matched for sex, age, and weight. A list of subject characteristics and results for strength and endurance is provided in Table 1. Unfortunately, we did not test the control subjects for perceptions of effort; instead, comparison data from the study of young healthy adults were used (Somodi et al., submitted).

MRS. S.

Pertinent History and Neurologic Examination

Mrs. S., a 65-year-old ambidextrous woman, was diagnosed with idiopathic Parkinson's disease on September 13, 1991. At that time, her neurologist assessed the disease severity as mild (Stage 2 on the Hoehn and Yahr scale, 1967). Levodopa-carbidopa (25/100, t.i.d.) and vitamin E were prescribed. Mrs. S. reported no change in either her speech or facial expression since the onset of parkinsonian symptoms in the left arm 2 years earlier.

Initial Evaluation

Our evaluation on the same day (9/13/91, before medications were taken) revealed moderately masked facial expression and mild-to-moderate hypokinetic dysarthria. Her voice was markedly monopitch, speech rate during a picture description task was fast (5.62 syllables/sec, with pauses excluded), phrases produced on one breath were long, and articulation was mildly imprecise. These characteristics are consistent with mild-to-moderate hypokinetic dysarthria. The matched-control subject's speech was normal, and her interpause speech rate was 4.79 syllables/sec.

Evaluations of tongue and hand strength and endurance were conducted. Using the IOPI protocol, maximum tongue pressure was 70 kPa and maximum right hand pressure was 112 kPa. Endurance at 50% of the maximum pressure was 45 sec for the tongue and 83 sec for the right hand. These data are comparable to those for the matched-control subject whose tongue strength was 53 kPa, hand strength was 169 kPa, tongue endurance was 43 sec, and hand endurance was 60 sec. In addition, Mrs. S.'s strength measures were similar to, and endurance measures were better than, those obtained from neurologically normal women of the same age (Lorell, Robin, et al., 1992). We concluded from this evaluation that,

Table 1. Subject characteristics and test results

Subject	Age (yrs)	Weight (kg)	Strength		Endurance		Speech rate (syllables/sec)	Overall speech
			tongue (kPa)	hand (kPa)	tongue (sec)	hand (sec)		
Mrs. S.								
Eval. 1	65	79.1	70	112	45	83	5.62	mild-to-moderate
Eval. 2			77	129	54	31[a]	5.14	mild-to-moderate
Control	64	77.7	53	169	43	60	4.79	normal
Mrs. H.								
Eval. 1	71	55.4	29	149	19; 55[b]	52	4.98	mild
Eval. 2			27	137	9[c]	55	5.03	mild
Control	72	55.0	50	126	32	30	5.27	normal
Mr. N.								
Eval. 1	43	92.2	53	273	6	14	4.23	mild
Eval. 2			39	239	18	39	3.36	mild
Control	45	92.2	70	156	25	24	5.44	normal

[a]Mrs. S. terminated the task early because of generalized fatigue.

[b]Tongue endurance task was repeated because Mrs. H. had difficulty controlling the pressure with her tongue.

[c]Mrs. H. appeared to have trouble controlling the pressure in this task.

although Mrs. S. exhibited mild Parkinson's disease and mild-to-moderate hypokinetic dysarthria, she had normal strength and endurance of the tongue and hand.

Follow-Up Evaluation

We evaluated Mrs. S. again on 1/31/92. Testing began four hours after her morning dose of levodopa-carbidopa. Similar speech characteristics as those observed during the initial session were noted. Maximum tongue strength was 77 kPa, and hand strength was 129 kPa. Endurance was 54 sec for the tongue. Mrs. S. maintained 50% of maximum pressure with the hand for 31 sec, but admitted to terminating the task early due to generalized fatigue. Endurance was tested at the end of this one-hour session. Except for hand endurance, these results are similar to those obtained during the initial evaluation.

Before the endurance tests were conducted, perceptions of various levels of effort were assessed using the protocol described by Somodi et al. (submitted) and summarized previously. The results from one trial with the tongue are plotted in Figure 1A and for the hand in Figure 1B. For the tongue, the pressures exerted generally increased with increasing effort levels, but the pattern was more scattered than is typically seen for normal subjects (Somodi et al., submitted). The data are even more variable for the hand, indicating little relation between pressure and effort, except at the lowest effort levels. Interestingly, for both the tongue and hand, the pressures tended to be in the lower portion of the total range available. Neurologically normal young adults used a wider range of the available pressures for this task (20%–90%), and exerted relatively high pressures when asked to use high levels of effort (Somodi et al., submitted). Thus, although strength and endurance measures were normal, the perception of effort appeared to be abnormal.

MRS. H.

Pertinent History and Neurologic Examination

Mrs. H., a 71-year-old right-handed woman, was diagnosed with idiopathic Parkinson's disease in May 1988. On November 19, 1991, her neurologist assessed the severity of disease as mild-to-moderate (Stage 2.5 on the Hoehn and Yahr scale, 1967). Mrs. H., an avid tennis player for 20 years, recently had to reduce her activity level. Mrs. H. reported that her speech is a little slower and quieter than it used to be.

Initial Evaluation

Mrs. H. was evaluated on November 19, 1991. She had taken a dose of levodopa-carbidopa (either 25/100 or control-release 50/200; this infor-

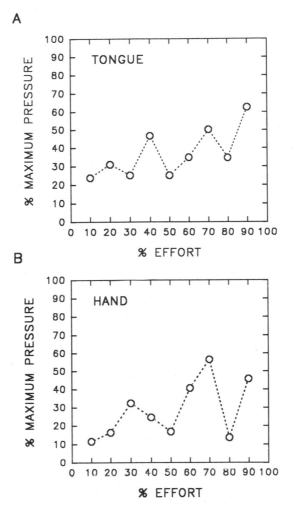

Figure 1. Effort results for Mrs. S. Pressures produced as a percentage of maximum pressure for various levels of effort for the tongue (A) and hand (B). Maximum pressure: tongue = 70 kPa, hand = 112 KPa.

mation was unavailable because Mrs. H. was a subject in a double-blind medication study) 2 hours and 40 minutes before testing. Her speech intelligibility was excellent, although mild articulatory imprecision was noted. Inconsistent vocal fry was perceived in her voice. Interpause speech rate was 4.98 syllables/sec. The control subject's speech was normal and speech rate was 5.27 syllables/sec.

Maximum tongue strength was 29 kPa, and maximum hand strength was 149 kPa. Endurance at 50% of maximum pressure was 19 sec, and 55 sec on a second trial, for the tongue, and 52 sec for the hand. The tongue endurance task was repeated because Mrs. H. had difficulty controlling the pressure with her tongue. The matched-control subject's tongue strength was 50 kPa, hand strength was 126 kPa, tongue endurance was 32 sec, and hand endurance was 30 sec. The control-subject's values, with the exception of hand endurance, which was reduced, were similar to data from other women of this age (Lorell, Robin, et al., 1992). Mrs. H.'s strength and endurance were normal for the hand; however, tongue strength was markedly reduced compared to normal, and tongue endurance times were variable.

Follow-Up Evaluation

We reevaluated Mrs. H. for tongue and hand function on March 4, 1992. Mrs. H. reported worsening of motor signs, now involving the left leg in addition to the previously affected right arm and leg. She did not notice a change in her speech.

Testing began 15 minutes after a dose of levodopa-carbidopa was taken. Her speech intelligibility, articulation, and speech rate were essentially unchanged from the initial session. However, the vocal fry was absent.

Maximum strength was 27 kPa for the tongue and 137 kPa for the hand. Mrs. H. was able to maintain 50% of maximum pressure with the tongue for only 9 sec, apparently because of difficulty controlling the pressure. Hand endurance was 55 sec. Except for tongue endurance, these findings are consistent with the initial evaluation.

Evaluation for the perception of various levels of effort revealed relatively typical findings for the hand, but markedly unusual findings for the tongue. The results are illustrated in Figure 2. Pressures exerted by the hand increased with increasing effort (Figure 2B). The results for the tongue appear to be almost random (Figure 2A). It should be noted that, for both the tongue and the hand, most pressures exerted are relatively high. Based on the results of this evaluation, it seems Mrs. H. has significant difficulty controlling and monitoring tongue movements for non-speech tasks. However, her speech was very good and might not have been affected by these abnormalities.

MR. N.

Pertinent History and Neurologic Examination

Mr. N., a 43-year-old left-handed man, reported difficulty with movement on the right side of the body in April 1988. In February 1991, he was diagnosed with parkinsonism that was considered to be secondary for etiology because of a history of drug abuse (meperidine hydrochloride).

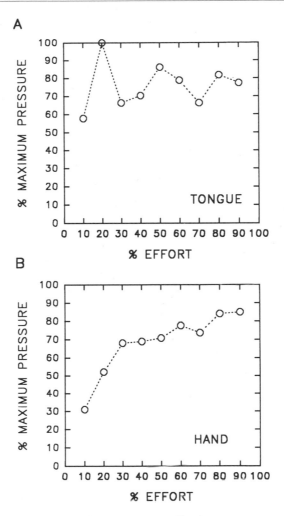

Figure 2. Effort results for Mrs. H. for the tongue (A) and hand (B). Maximum pressure: tongue = 31 KPa, hand = 149 KPa.

One year after diagnosis (1/31/92), his neurologist described the disease severity as mild-to-moderate (Stage 2.5, Hoehn & Yahr, 1967), and Mr. N. was on disability leave from his job as a warehouse worker. Mr. N. reported that his speech was mildly affected; vocal intensity decreased progressively during running speech, and some "slurring" occurred.

Initial Evaluation

We evaluated Mr. N. for tongue function and speech on January 31, 1992. He took levodopa-carbidopa (25/250) 4 hours and 30 minutes before testing. His speech was completely intelligible, interpause speech rate was slow (4.23 syllables/sec), and voice quality was breathy. The matched-control subject had normal speech and an interpause speech rate of 5.44 syllables/sec.

Tongue strength was assessed at 53 kPa, and left hand strength was 273 kPa. Endurance at 50% maximum pressure was 6 sec for the tongue and 14 sec for the hand. The matched-control subject's tongue strength was 70 kPa, preferred (left) hand strength was 156 kPa, tongue endurance was 25 sec, and hand endurance was 24 sec. The control subject's data are typical for men his age, with the exception of markedly reduced hand endurance (Lorell, Robin, et al., 1992). These data reveal that Mr. N.'s tongue strength was somewhat lower than normal, hand strength was much greater than normal, and endurance times for both the tongue and hand were substantially reduced.

Follow-Up Evaluation

One month later (2/25/92), 3 hours after a dose of levodopa-carbidopa, Mr. N. was re-evaluated. His speech was notably impaired. Intelligibility was still excellent, but monotony of pitch and loudness were pervasive, and interpause speech rate was markedly slower (3.36 syllables/sec). Voice quality was similarly breathy.

Tongue strength was determined to be 39 kPa and hand strength 239 kPa. Both these values are lower than those from the initial evaluation. Endurance at 50% maximum pressure was 18 sec for the tongue and 39 sec for the hand. Although these endurance times are somewhat better than those obtained previously (possibly because the maximum pressures were lower), they remain abnormally brief.

The pressure-effort relationship for the hand (Figure 3B) was relatively linear with pressure increasing with effort. The function is similar to that obtained from healthy young subjects, except that the pressures exerted at the effort extremes were restricted to the middle of the pressure range (33%–70%) rather than showing the usual sensitivity to pressure differences. The findings for the tongue are quite unusual (Figure 3A). There does not appear to be a systematic relationship between effort and pressure. Most attempts at various effort levels resulted in pressures of approximately 60%–80% of the tongue's maximum pressure. Exceptions to this general finding are bizarre—Mr. N. exerted 96% of his maximum pressure when asked to give 60% effort, and 38% of maximum pressure for 80% effort.

The results from Mr. N.'s follow-up evaluation confirm that tongue strength and endurance were abnormally reduced, and suggest that he has little awareness of actual pressures exerted by his tongue. It is tempting to speculate that Mr. N.'s abnormally slow speech rate may be related to

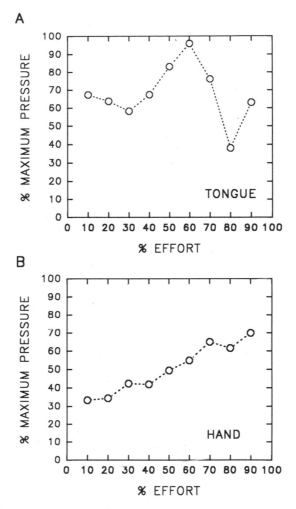

Figure 3. Effort results for Mr. N. for the tongue (A) and hand (B). Maximum pressure: tongue = 39 KPa, hand = 239 KPa.

these abnormalities. This notion is supported by the decrease in both speech rate and tongue strength from the first to the second session.

SUMMARY

The relations between strength, endurance, and perceptions of effort are unclear. Our ultimate goal is to assess these features of motor control in the tongue and to determine their relation to speech characteristics. Previous evaluations of tongue strength and endurance in a variety of normal and disordered populations have provided interesting clinical and basic information. The technique for the study of effort perceptions, described by Somodi et al. (submitted), was added recently to the standard evaluation procedures. This measure may reveal clues for the explanation of abnormally low endurance levels and symptoms of fatigue during speech.

In this chapter, we presented case studies of three people with mild parkinsonism and symptoms of generalized fatigue. Our results provide intriguing patterns of findings. Two profiles are particularly interesting. First, one subject, Mrs. S., had normal strength and endurance in the tongue and hand, but her perceptions of effort were abnormal. Besides the marked variability in her responses to the effort task, the pressures produced were relatively low, even at high levels of effort. This finding is consistent with Mrs. S.'s general perception of fatigue. Second, the two subjects with low strength and low or abnormally variable endurance of the tongue (Mrs. H. and Mr. N.) exhibited abnormally variable responses to the effort task and produced pressures near their maximum strength across the effort range. Typically, individuals with weakened muscles have an increased sense of effort (Gandevia, 1982; McCloskey, 1981), which may explain these results. Because of low tongue strength, they may perceive a need to produce near maximal pressures to accomplish tasks of any effort level.

The tongue function evaluation involves nonspeech tasks, and their relation to speech proficiency is unknown. Based on these three cases and a previous investigation, we can speculate that tongue endurance may correlate with speech rate. In the present report, Mrs. S. had normal tongue endurance and a fast speech rate, and Mr. N. had low tongue endurance and a slow speech rate. Similarly, neurologically normal speakers with fast speech rates had better than normal tongue endurance (Robin et al., 1992). Following this logic, we would have expected Mr. N.'s tongue endurance to be better when his speech rate was faster, but this did not occur. Obviously, these preliminary observations are insufficient for drawing conclusions about speech rate and tongue endurance. Another puzzling finding was that Mrs. H.'s speech rate and intelligibility were normal, yet all three tongue function tests were abnormal. Perhaps the abnormalities were too mild to affect speech, or Mrs. H. was able to compensate successfully for these impairments. These results reinforce the need for further investigation into the relation between speech and nonspeech tongue function measures.

We are beginning to study a larger group of people with Parkinson's disease, especially those in more advanced stages of the disease, using a similar protocol for tongue function testing. We shall examine tongue function in terms of the relations between strength, endurance, and effort, and the correlations between these features and specific speech characteristics. Ultimately, we hope to understand fatigue better and to learn how to cope with it in the management of individuals with neuromotor speech disorders.

REFERENCES

Canter, G.J. (1965). Speech characteristics of patients with Parkinson's disease: III. Articulation, diadochokinesis, and over-all speech adequacy. *Journal of Speech and Hearing Disorders, 30,* 217–224.

Darley, F.L., Aronson, A.E., & Brown, J.R. (1975). *Motor speech disorders.* Philadelphia: W.B. Saunders.

Edwards, R.H.T. (1981). Human muscle function and fatigue. In R. Porter & J. Whelan (Eds.), *Human muscle fatigue: Physiological mechanisms* (pp. 1–18). London: Pitman Medical.

Enoka, R.M., & Stuart, D.G. (1985). The contribution of neuroscience to exercise studies. *Federation Proceedings, 44,* 2279–2285.

Gandevia, S.C. (1982). The perception of motor commands or effort during muscular paralysis. *Brain, 105,* 151–159.

Goodglass, H., & Kaplan, E. (1981). *The assessment of aphasia and related disorders* (2nd ed.). Philadelphia: Lea & Febiger.

Hoehn, M.M., & Yahr, M.D. (1967). Parkinsonism: Onset, progression, and mortality. *Neurology, 17,* 427–442.

Logemann, J.A., Fisher, H.B., Boshes, B., & Blonsky, E.R. (1978). Frequency and co-occurrence of vocal tract dysfunctions in the speech of a large sample of Parkinson patients. *Journal of Speech and Hearing Disorders, 43,* 47–57.

Lorell, D.M., Robin, D.A., Somodi, L.B., Solomon, N.P., & Luschei, E.S. (1992, November). Tongue strength and endurance in the elderly. *Asha* (Abstract), *34,* 175.

Lorell, D.M., Solomon, N.P., Robin, D.A., Somodi, L.B., Rodnitzky, R., & Luschei, E.S. (1992, April). *Tongue strength and endurance in individuals with Parkinson's disease.* Paper presented at the Conference on Motor Speech, Boulder, CO.

Mayeux, R., Stern, Y., Williams, J.B.W., Cote, J., Frantz, A., & Dyrenfurth, I. (1986). Clinical and biochemical features of depression in Parkinson's disease. *American Journal of Psychiatry, 143,* 756–759.

McCloskey, D.I. (1981). Corollary discharges: Motor commands and perception. In V.B. Brooks (Ed.), *Handbook of physiology: Sect. 1, Vol. II, The nervous system: Motor control, Part 2* (pp. 1415–1447). Bethesda, MD: American Physiological Society.

McDowell, F.H. (1971). The diagnosis of parkinsonism or Parkinson syndrome. In F.H. McDowell & C.H. Markham (Eds.), *Recent advances in Parkinson's disease* (pp. 163–174). Philadelphia: F.A. Davis Co.

Neilson, P.D., & O'Dwyer, N.J. (1984). Reproducibility and variability of speech muscle activity in athetoid dysarthria of cerebral palsy. *Journal of Speech and Hearing Research, 27,* 502–517.

Robin, D.A., Goel, A., Somodi, L.B., & Luschei, E.S. (1992). Tongue strength and endurance: Relation to highly skilled movements. *Journal of Speech and Hearing Research, 35,* 1239–1245.

Robin, D.A., Somodi, L.B., & Luschei, E.S. (1991). Measurement of tongue strength and endurance in normal and articulation disordered subjects. In C.A. Moore, K.M. Yorkston, & D.R. Beukelman (Eds.), *Dysarthria and apraxia of speech: Perspectives on management* (pp. 173–184). Baltimore: Paul H. Brookes Publishing Co.

Solomon, N.P., & Hixon, T.J. (1993). Speech breathing in Parkinson's disease. *Journal of Speech and Hearing Research, 36,* 294–310.

Solomon, N.P., Lorell, D.M., Robin, D.A., Rodnitzky, R.L., & Luschei, E.S. (submitted). *Tongue strength and endurance in mild to moderate Parkinson's disease.*

Somodi, L.B., Robin, D.A., & Luschei, E.S. (submitted). *A model of "sense of effort" during maximal and submaximal contractions of the tongue.*

Chapter 12

Effect of Instruction on Selected Aerodynamic Parameters in Subjects with Dysarthria and Control Subjects

Vicki L. Hammen and Kathryn M. Yorkston

MEASURES OF UPPER vocal tract aerodynamics can be useful in assessment of the motor speech performance of individuals with dysarthria. Intra-oral air pressure and nasal airflow have been used to evaluate velopharyngeal function in speakers with dysarthria (Netsell, 1969; Yorkston, Beukelman, Honsinger, & Mitsuda, 1989). These measures can document the nature and extent of the impairment and can guide certain intervention approaches, such as palatal lift fittings. Until recently, however, extensive instrumentation and time-consuming analyses limited clinical use of such measures. Development of computer-based analysis systems (Barlow, Suing, Grossman, Bodmer, & Colbert, 1989) that streamline the computational aspects of physiologic measurements will enable clinicians to obtain physiologic data on their patients with dysarthria. However, as more clinical centers that evaluate and manage individuals with dysarthria begin to incorporate these types of measures into their assessment protocols, standardization of stimuli becomes critical. The influence of instruction on a subject's performance must be evaluated as part of the development of standardized assessment protocols.

This work was supported in part by Grant No. H133B80081 from the National Institute on Disability and Rehabilitation Research, Department of Education, Washington, D.C. This work is in the public domain.

Instruction has been shown to alter the performance of subjects on selected speech tasks. Picheny and colleagues (Picheny, Durlach, & Braida, 1985, 1986, 1989) examined the effects of instructing individuals to speak as clearly as possible on several parameters with hearing-impaired listeners. Intelligibility, speaking rate, and phonetic characteristics were all altered during the instruction period. Moreover, Reich, Mason, and Polen (1986) found increases in maximum phonation time when subjects received instruction and coaching.

In addition to the issue of standardized stimuli presentation, the response to instruction is an important component in the assessment process of individuals with dysarthria (Yorkston, Beukelman, & Bell, 1988). Most clinicians agree that the ability of a speaker with dysarthria to modify productions when instructed to do so is a positive prognostic indicator. However, little information is available regarding the ability of such a speaker to modify speech production. Therefore, this study was conducted to examine the effect of instruction on selected aerodynamic parameters of speech production. The following questions were posed during this investigation. First, do subjects with dysarthria and control subjects modify their performances in response to instruction? Second, does within task variability change as a function of instruction in subjects with dysarthria and control subjects? Finally, how many tokens are needed in order to obtain a representative sample of mean performance and variability?

METHOD

Subjects

Fourteen individuals with dysarthria, seven males and seven females, were subjects. They were solicited from the clinical population served by Speech Pathology Services at the University of Washington Medical Center, Seattle. Their ages ranged from 19 to 53 years with a mean of 30 years. Ten subjects were diagnosed with traumatic brain injury (TBI), three with cerebral vascular accident (CVA), and one with amyotrophic lateral sclerosis (ALS). The majority were highly intelligible, with 10 subjects greater than 90% intelligible and 4 less than 90% intelligible, as tested on the sentence portion of the Computerized Assessment of Intelligibility of Dysarthric Speech (Yorkston, Beukelman, & Traynor, 1984). The primary perceptual characteristic of the dysarthria was determined by the clinician responsible for the evaluation and treatment of the patient, and was confirmed by the senior author. Nine subjects were characterized by an ataxic dysarthria, three mixed, and two a flaccid dysarthria. Cognitive status for the individuals with traumatic brain injury was at or above Level VII on the Rancho Scale (Hagen, 1984).

Seven non-neurologically impaired speakers with American English as their primary language and no history of speech problems were selected as control subjects. They were chosen to correspond to the age and gender distribution of the subjects with dysarthria. There were three male and four female control subjects whose ages ranged from 20 to 46 years, with a mean of 31 years.

Data Acquisition

Two measures were obtained during the course of this study, intra-oral air pressure and duration. The Speech Physiology Protocol Display System (Barlow et al., 1989) interfaced with an IBM 286-type computer was used to record the physiologic signals. Four channels of analog signals were acquired during data acquisition: intra-oral air pressure; nasal airflow; audio; and a token tag used during the analysis phase. Several data channels were recorded during data acquisition; however, this study focused solely on the intra-oral air pressure signal. To obtain air pressure data, a length of polyethylene tubing connected to a Statham pressure transducer (PM131TC) was inserted in the oral angle and placed perpendicular to the airflow, just behind the front teeth. The signals were bridge amplified and low-pass filtered at 50 Hz (Biocommunications Electronics) prior to digitization (R.C. Electronics ISC-16).

Task

Subjects repeated the phrase "Buy a puppy," 10 times during a habitual performance and two instructed performances. The habitual performance was always completed first during the experimental session. Prior to the habitual performance, subjects were told: "You will be saying a phrase 10 times while this mask is placed over your nose and this tube is placed inside your mouth, just behind your front teeth." Following each third production, subjects were told how many tokens remained before the task was complete. This was done to keep the task structure consistent with the instructed performances. Following the habitual performance, two instructed performances were presented in counterbalanced order. One solicited precise and the other forceful productions.

Subjects were given the following directions: "You will be saying 'Buy a puppy' 10 times, but this time I want you to say it as precisely/forcefully as you can. Make the 'p' and 'b' sounds as clear and precise as you possibly can [for the precise condition]" or "Really pop the 'p' and 'b' sounds a forcefully as possible [for the forceful condition]." Following each third production, subjects were re-instructed to say "Buy a puppy" as precisely/

forcefully as they could. This was done to minimize any memory demands of the task.

Signal Analysis

The digitized signals were analyzed using the AEROSPEECH software program (Barlow & Suing, 1992). This program provides the user with a graphic display of intra-oral air pressure, nasal airflow, and velopharyngeal resistance versus time for each recorded token. In addition, a separate file is created during analysis from which the value for each intra-oral air pressure peak can be obtained. A cursoring function allows the user to set cursors at specific points on the waveform and read the time between marked points from the computer screen.

Peak intra-oral air pressure in cm H_2O was taken from the first plosive in the word "puppy," which eliminated variation in the data due to voicing and/or stress. Phrase duration was defined for the purposes of this study as the time from the onset of intra-oral air pressure for the /b/ in "Buy" to the offset of pressure for the second /p/ in "puppy." Twenty percent of the data were re-displayed and analyzed to determine intra-judge reliability for the phrase duration measure. A correlation of 0.99 was obtained, indicating excellent reliability for this measure.

RESULTS AND DISCUSSION

Response to Instruction

Our first question was: Do subjects with dysarthria and control subjects modify their performances in response to instruction? In order to answer this, pressure and phrase duration data were averaged across speakers in the group with dysarthria and the control group. Figure 1 is a scatter plot of these data for the habitual, precise, and forceful performances.

A two-way repeated measure analysis of variance (groups by performance) was completed for each measure. Results for pressure showed a significant group effect ($F = .120; p = .73$) and no significant interaction between group and performances ($F = .328; p = .722$). The effect of performances was significant ($F = 19.335; p = .000$), with post hoc testing confirming the forceful performance was different from both the habitual and precise. Results for phrase duration showed a significant group effect ($F = .4.37; p = .05$), but no significant performance effect ($F = 1.523; p = .231$) or interaction between group and performances ($F = .328; p = .722$). Thus, speakers with dysarthria tended to produce longer phrase duration than control speakers. Both groups tend to modify their performances in response to instruction. When asked to produce an utterance more forcefully, both groups tended to increase intra-oral pressure. Al-

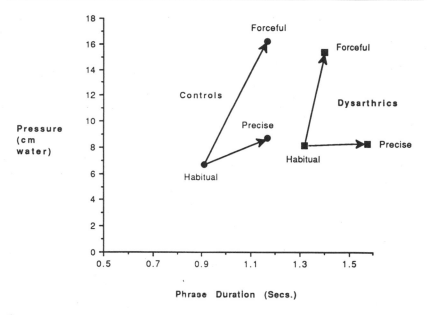

Figure 1. A scatterplot of mean intra-oral pressure and phrase duration data from control subjects and speakers with dysarthria. Habitual performance is compared with performance when subjects were asked to produce utterances either precisely or forcefully.

though Figure 1 suggests a trend toward lengthening in response to instruction, this trend was not statistically significant.

Within Task Variability

The second question was: Does within task variability change as a function of instruction? In order to answer this, coefficients of variation (CV) were computed for each speaker. CV was chosen rather than standard deviation (SD) as an index of variability because the magnitude of the SD can be expected to vary as a function of the magnitude of the mean. CV is calculated by dividing the SD by the mean. Figure 2 illustrates the mean CV for pressure and phrase duration in each of the conditions. This figure suggests a tendency for increased variability in the pressure measure during the forceful performance for both subjects with dysarthria and control subjects.

In order to explore changes in variability of intra-oral pressure measure as a function of instruction, data from individual subjects are plotted in Figure 3, which depicts the range of intra-oral air pressures for each performance. Note that during the habitual performance, ranges were small for the control group and somewhat larger and more variable for the group with dysarthria. It should be noted also that some speakers with

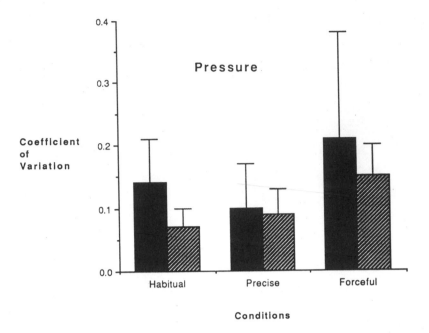

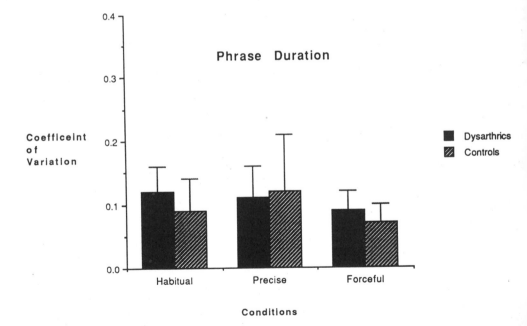

Figure 2. Coefficients of variation for the performance of subjects with dysarthria and control subjects on measures of intra-oral pressure and phrase duration. Three performances are shown—habitual, precise, and forceful.

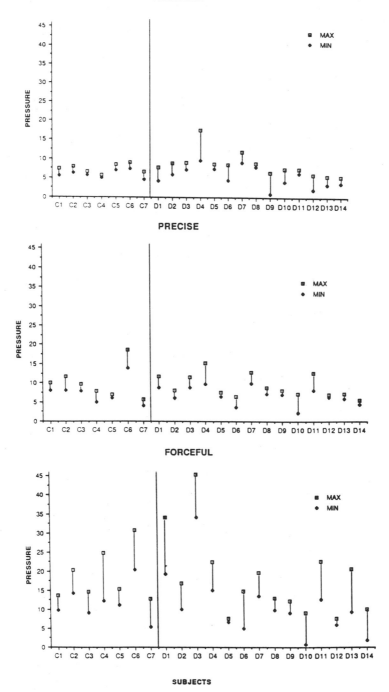

Figure 3. Maximum and minimum intra-oral air pressures for the control subjects (C) and the subjects with dysarthria (D) during habitual, precise, and forceful performances.

dysarthria displayed a range consistent with controls, whereas others did not. In the forceful performance, substantially larger ranges of intra-oral air pressure are observed for both groups. Again, some speakers with dysarthria showed larger ranges than the controls, whereas others exhibited ranges smaller than the controls.

A final method of characterizing the variability of subjects is shown in Figure 4. Z-scores were calculated and plotted for pressure and duration for each subject during the habitual performance. If a subject's data were exactly at the mean value obtained from the control group for both pressure and duration, the data point would be at the zero-zero location. Vertical and horizontal reference lines have been placed at the +1 and −1 standard deviation point for pressure and duration, respectively. From this figure, it seems that both groups tended to vary primarily along the pressure dimension, with little variation along the durational axis. Most subjects would fall within a +2 or −2 standard deviation range on this task. The only subjects outside this range were in the group with dysarthria, and were identified in both measures.

Examination of individual data thus far has suggested the potential for large variability in performance for some speakers. This variability is of concern in the clinical examination setting where the goal is to characterize performance, but to do so rapidly and efficiently. Our final question

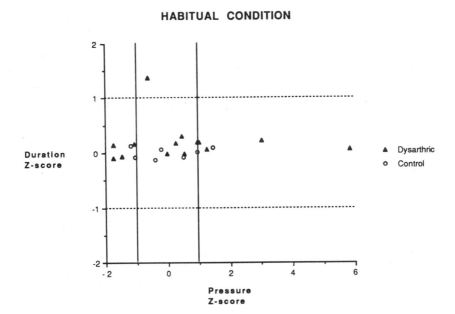

Figure 4. Z-scores for phrase duration and intra-oral air pressure for both groups.

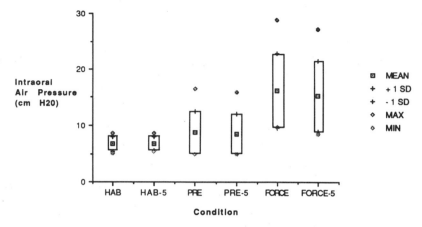

Figure 5. Central tendency statistics for intra-oral air pressure for the habitual (HAB), precise (PRE), and forceful (FORCE) performances averaged across all 10 tokens versus the first 5 tokens (HAB-5, PRE-5, FORCE-5) for the control subjects.

was: How many tokens are required to obtain a representative sample of mean performance and variability? To answer this, the descriptive statistics from the first 5 tokens were compared with those obtained from the entire set of 10 tokens. The results are shown in Figure 5 for the control subjects and in Figure 6 for the subjects with dysarthria. For both groups, the difference between the mean intra-oral air pressure from the first 5 tokens and the total of 10 tokens averaged 0.78 cm H_2O, with a range of 0.04 to 3.18 cm H_2O. Therefore, it seems that five tokens were sufficient to characterize both habitual and instructed performance on this task.

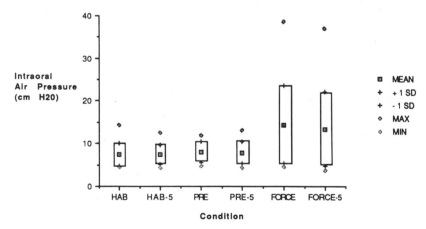

Figure 6. Central tendency statistics for intra-oral air pressure (in cm H_2O) for the habitual (HAB), precise (PRE), and forceful (FORCE) performances averaged across all 10 tokens versus the first 5 tokens (HAB-5, PRE-5, FORCE-5) for the control subjects.

Finally, although there are several ways to characterize the group data, some interesting performance patterns demonstrated by individual subjects could be lost when means are presented. Figures 7 and 8 show the results for intra-oral air pressure and phrase duration for two particularly interesting cases. Both subjects had a diagnosis of traumatic brain injury and were highly intelligible. As shown in Figure 7, both had similar intra-

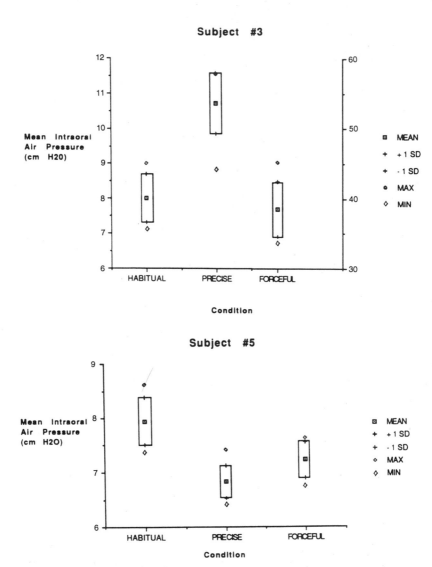

Figure 7. Central tendency statistics for intra-oral air pressure (in cm H$_2$O) for two individual subjects with dysarthria (#3 and #5).

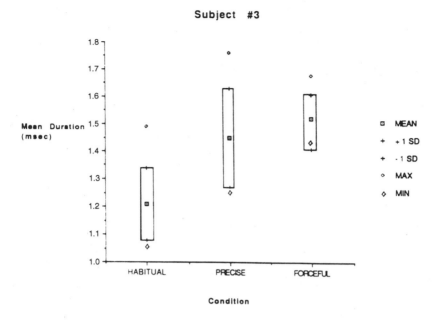

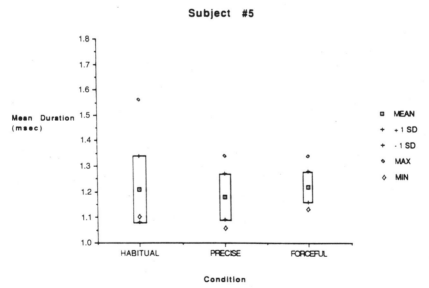

Figure 8. Central tendency statistics for phrase duration (milliseconds) for two individual subjects with dysarthria (#3 and #5).

oral air pressures, around 8 cm H_2O, during the habitual performance. Yet, when instructed to be precise, subject three increased pressure (to

10.71 cm H_2O), while subject five actually decreased intra-oral air pressure (to 6.83 cm H_2O). During the forceful performance, subject three produced an average of 38.55 cm H_2O pressure (scale on the right side of the figure). Subject five again slightly decreased pressure relative to the habitual performance (7.23 cm H_2O).

Similar trends were observed when duration was examined (Figure 8). Both subjects produced the phrase in 1.2 msec during the habitual performance. Subject five demonstrated little change in duration across the two instructed performances (1.18 msec and 1.22 msec for the precise and forceful performances, respectively). Subject three showed increases in duration for both precise and forceful performances (1.45 msec and 1.52 msec for the precise and forceful performances, respectively). However, both subjects showed a reduction in variability during the forceful performance, similar to the group findings.

CLINICAL IMPLICATIONS

Clinicians frequently make decisions about treatment candidacy based on their impressions of a subject's ability to modify habitual production. A long-term goal of this research is to use measures of selected aerodynamic aspects of speech production to serve not only as objective measures of habitual performance, but combined with other measures, to provide insight into a speakers' ability to respond to intervention. The results of this study indicated that many, but not all, subjects modified their performances in response to instruction. They showed similar tendencies when they modified speech production; that is, pressure was increased significantly in the forceful performance. Variability was increased when subjects were instructed to produce the utterance forcefully. This suggests that some subjects were able to change speech production characteristics in response to instruction, whereas others were not; therefore, habitual performance might be more stable than instructed performance. Five tokens seemed adequate to characterize subject performance on these tasks. Caution is warranted when interpreting group data. Such data may not be representative of individual subject performance, even when subjects are similar in etiology and severity of dysarthria. Until we have a better understanding of the nature of the underlying physiologic impairment in groups of speakers with dysarthria, clinicians must continue to view each individual with dysarthria as unique with varying habitual performance and varying ability to modify that performance.

REFERENCES

Barlow, S.M., & Suing, G. (1992). AEROSPEECH: Automated digital signal analysis of speech aerodynamics. *Journal of Computer Users in Speech and Hearing*, 7, 211–227.

Barlow, S.M., Suing, G., Grossman, A., Bodmer, P., & Colbert, R. (1989). A high-speed data-acquisition and protocol system for vocal tract physiology. *Journal of Voice, 3*, 283–293.

Hagen, C. (1984). Language disorders in head trauma. In A. Holland (Ed.), *Language disorders in adults: Recent advances* (pp. 245–282). Austin, TX: PRO-ED.

Netsell, R. (1969). Evaluation of velopharyngeal function in dysarthria. *Journal of Speech and Hearing Disorders, 34*, 113–122.

Picheny, M., Durlach, N., & Braida, L. (1985). Speaking clearly for the hard of hearing I: Intelligibility differences between clear and conversational speech. *Journal of Speech and Hearing Research, 28*, 96–103.

Picheny, M., Dulach, N., & Braida, L. (1986). Speaking clearly for the hard of hearing II: Acoustic characteristics of clear and conversational speech. *Journal of Speech and Hearing Research, 29*, 434–446.

Picheny, M., Durlach, N., & Braida, L. (1989). Speaking clearly for the hard of hearing III: An attempt to determine the contribution of speaking rate to differences in intelligibility between clear and conversational speech. *Journal of Speech and Hearing Research, 32*, 600–603.

Reich, A.R., Mason, J.A., & Polen, S.B. (1986). Task administration variables affecting phonation-time measures in third grade girls with normal voice quality. *Language, Speech and Hearing Services in Schools, 17*, 262–269.

Yorkston, K.M., Beukelman, D.R., & Bell, K.R. (1988). *Clinical management of dysarthric speakers.* Austin, TX: PRO-ED.

Yorkston, K.M., Beukelman, D.R., & Traynor, C. (1984). *Computerized assessment of intelligibility of dysarthric speech.* Austin, TX: PRO-ED.

Yorkston, K.M., Beukelman, D.R., Honsinger, M.J., & Mitsuda, P.A. (1989). Perceived articulatory adequacy and velopharyngeal function in dysarthric speakers. *Archives of Physical Medicine and Rehabilitation, 70*, 313–317.

Chapter 13

Semantic Context and Speech Intelligibility

Paul A. Dongilli, Jr.

CONTEXT CAN PLAY an active role in a listener's ability to discriminate or perceive a distorted or imprecise speech signal. The notion of context as a factor influencing an individual's speech intelligibility implies interaction between the speaker and listener. This concept has been explored recently in detail by Lindblom (1990), who referred to it as "mutuality."

The premise underlying Lindblom's (1990) mutuality model is that speech intelligibility is not determined exclusively by the quality of the speech signal. Listener knowledge has an impact on the intelligibility of imprecise or distorted signals as well. Specifically, linguistic knowledge, language redundancy, and contextual knowledge allow listeners to discriminate incomplete or distorted messages. Signal information and listener knowledge (signal-independent information) serve complementary roles and interact to result in successful communication. For purposes of this discussion, listener knowledge is viewed as the context of the signal or message. The mutuality model predicts that signal "rich" or high quality information can be perceived readily in light of signal-independent information (context) that is "poor," or absent. As the signal information deteriorates or becomes poor, the signal-independent information, or context, must be enhanced or enriched for intelligibility to be deemed high. Highly distorted, or poor signal information, in conjunction with absent or poor signal-independent information results in the perception of low intelligibility.

It is clear from the mutuality model that speech intelligibility can be influenced by two major factors—the speech signal itself, and the message context. This context is composed of the syntactic and semantic knowl-

175

edge of the listener. Therefore, knowledge regarding the syntactic and semantic context of a message has the potential to affect speech intelligibility greatly.

The effects of utterance length (words versus sentences) on speech intelligibility have been documented in individuals with speech intelligibility disorders secondary to hearing impairment and dysarthria (McGarr, 1981; 1983; Sitler, Schiavetti, & Metz, 1983; Yorkston & Beukelman, 1978). This literature reveals that providing listeners with sentence length utterances results in increased speech intelligibility. Furthermore, there is an interaction between utterance length and severity of the intelligibility impairment, with the influence of utterance length resulting in greater intelligibility scores for sentences when overall intelligibility is above 20%–30%. When intelligibility scores are below 20%–30%, single word intelligibility scores are greater than scores for sentences.

Although semantic context is an inherent component of syntactic context, only preliminary studies of semantic context on the intelligibility of dysarthric speech have been reported. Semantic context can be defined as contextual cues that suggest a topic or setting in which a word or sentence may have been uttered (Monsen, 1983). Hammen, Yorkston, and Dowden (1991) documented the positive effects of semantic context on the intelligibility of production of single words in speakers with dysarthria. These speakers were selected to represent a spectrum of intelligibility impairment ranging from moderate to profound. Interaction between context and severity of dysarthric speech was observed, with the greatest intelligibility improvements noted for the severe group, intermediate improvements recorded for the moderate group, and the lowest improvements noted for the profound group. In this study, the quality of the speech signal was not changed. Rather, a signal-independent factor, semantic context, was manipulated and it was this factor that contributed to the recorded improvements in speech intelligibility.

Improved intelligibility in the presence of semantic context was also documented in hearing-impaired individuals' production of sentences (Monsen, 1983). Signal-independent information was manipulated resulting in increased intelligibility. Based on the results of Monsen's study, it is tempting to generalize the positive effects of semantic context to the speech intelligibility of the sentences production of speakers with dysarthria. However, this enthusiasm should be restrained because speakers with dysarthria and hearing impairment may experience decreased speech intelligibility for different reasons. Furthermore, the type of contextual cues used in the two research studies differed. Monsen used sentence-length semantic contextual cues with hearing-impaired subjects whereas Hammen et al. (1991) used single-word category labels, most frequently single words. Thus, further research is needed to document the influence of utterance length and semantic context on the speech intelligibility of individuals with dysarthria and to determine the nature of the interaction between these factors and speech intelligibility.

METHOD

Subjects

The subjects in this study were two groups, eight speakers with dysarthria and 96 listeners.

Speakers with Dysarthria Eight individuals with primarily flaccid dysarthric were selected to reflect a severity range from mild to profound. Table 1 presents demographic information for these eight speakers, four females and four males, ranging in age from 23 to 87 years. Etiologies were traumatic brain injury (TBI) and cerebrovascular accident (CVA). No speaker with dysarthria had a developmental history of speech, language, hearing, or neurologic problems.

The speakers were primarily flaccid dysarthric speakers, according to the perceptual classification system outlined by Darley, Aronson, and Brown (1975). Three speech-language pathologists, familiar with dysarthric speech, confirmed independently that the speakers exhibited primarily flaccid dysarthria based on an analysis of a recorded sample of spontaneous speech.

Classification of dysarthric severity was based on a prestudy screening measure, which consisted of the single-word intelligibility subtest (Yorkston & Beukelman, 1981). Intelligibility scores were calculated using the transcriptional scoring format of this test battery. A single-word intelligibility score ranging from 0 to 25 resulted in the classification of profound; from 30 to 45 resulted in the classification of severe; from 50 to 65 resulted in the classification of moderate; and from 70 to 95 resulted in the

Table 1. Demographic information and word intelligibility scores

Subject	Age/gender	Diagnosis	Prescreening word intelligibility score (%)	Severity classification
1	87/M	CVA	54	Moderate
2	52/F	CVA	32	Severe
3	32/M	TBI	90	Mild
4	43/M	TBI	74	Mild
5	65/F	CVA	38	Severe
6	69/F	CVA	62	Moderate
7	71/M	CVA	0	Profound
8	23/F	TBI	8	Profound

classification of mild. At least a 10-point intelligibility score differentiated subjects between classification groups. Two speakers with dysarthria were selected for each of the four severity classifications.

Listeners Non–hearing disabled individuals between the ages of 19 and 50 years, who were not familiar with dysarthric speech or the stimulus materials, served as listeners. These individuals passed on audiometric, air conduction, pure tone screening at 25 db for the frequencies 500, 1000, 2000, and 4000 Hz. The listeners were assigned randomly to one of eight groups consisting of 12 listeners (96 listeners in all).

Stimulus Materials

Listening Tapes Each speaker with dysarthria read aloud four separate, shortened versions of the speech perception in noise (SPIN) test (Kalikow, Stevens, & Elliott, 1977). Stimulus items from this test were used in this study because they were designed to incorporate the linguistic-situational information of speech rather than acoustic-phonetic information only. From each test version, the speaker with dysarthria orally read either the 25 stimulus words in isolation or embedded within the high probability test sentences. Bigler (1984) outlined the measures taken to ensure equivalency of test versions for this test.

The readings were recorded in a quiet room with a UHER Model 4200/4400 tape recorder, using a Sennheiser Model K3N/K3U microphone positioned approximately 15 cm from the speaker's mouth. All recordings were completed in a single session. The speakers with dysarthria were instructed to read each word and sentence as they would normally. If any portion of the word or sentence was misread, that word or sentence was re-recorded in its entirety.

Eight listening tapes were constructed from these recordings. Each tape contained two sets of 25 single words and two sets of 25 sentences. Each tape was prepared so that each set of words and sentences was selected from a different test version of SPIN.

Semantic Contextual Cues Semantic contextual cues were developed for one set of words and one set of sentences used in the series of listening tapes in the following manner. Speech-language pathologists served as judges and were presented with all the words from the four test versions of SPIN used in this study. They were instructed to read each word and to list the category or context within which the word belonged. For example, the test word "swan" resulted in the generation of the semantic contextual cue of "bird." Following this procedure, the judges were presented with all the sentences from the four test versions of SPIN used in this study. They were instructed to read each sentence and to list the context or setting in which the sentence might have been uttered. For example, the test sentence, "The ducks swam around the pond," resulted in the generation of the semantic contextual cue of "park." Three of the four judges had to agree on the semantic context for each word and sentence for that context to be accepted as a semantic contextual cue. After reviewing the judges responses utilizing these criteria, acceptable semantic contextual cues were evident for only a single set of words and a single set of sentences, which were used for the word transcription with semantic context and the sentence transcription with semantic context measurement conditions.

Measurement Conditions

Four measurement conditions were developed for this study: 1) word transcription without semantic context, 2) word transcription with semantic context, 3) sentence transcription without semantic context, and 4) sentence transcription with semantic context.

Word Transcription without Semantic Context Listeners heard 25 words presented individually and were asked to transcribe each word orthographically as they heard it. (See Appendix A for the list of stimulus words.)

Word Transcription with Semantic Context Listeners heard 25 words presented individually and were asked to transcribe each word orthographically, as in the context described above. However, before hearing each word, the listeners were provided with a semantic contextual cue. Listeners were then instructed to answer, not solely on the basis of the cue, but rather, on the basis of the word combined with the cue. (See Appendix B for a list of stimulus words and semantic contextual cues.)

Sentence Transcription without Semantic Context Listeners heard each sentence and were asked to transcribe orthographically what they had heard. Listeners were permitted to hear the sentence a second time if a repetition was requested. (See Appendix C for the list of stimulus materials.)

Sentence Transcription with Semantic Context Listeners heard each sentence and were asked to transcribe orthographically what they had heard, as in the context above. However, before hearing each sentence, the listeners were provided with a semantic contextual cue. Listeners were then instructed to answer, not solely on the basis of the cue, but rather, on the basis of the sentence combined with the cue. (See Appendix D for a list of stimulus materials and semantic contextual cues.)

Procedures

Each speaker with dysarthria was paired randomly with a group of 12 listeners. The 12 listeners assigned to a speaker were divided into groups of three. The order of presentation of the stimulus material from the four conditions was counterbalanced for each listening group. The listeners transcribed the listening tapes of the speaker with dysarthria under all four conditions. All tapes were presented to the listeners on the TEAC X-300 tape recorder attached to a Realistic SA-150 integrated stereo amplifier and two Realistic minimus-18 speakers. The speakers were positioned approximately 24–36 inches from the listening group. Listening sessions were completed in a quiet room and transcribed in a single sitting. At least one week following completion of the initial transcriptions, 12 listeners were randomly selected from the pool of 96 listeners to retranscribe their respective samples as an intrajudge reliability measure. The responses obtained for the original and reliability transcriptions for each listener were compared on a point-by-point basis. Agreement was confirmed if the transcription of the stimulus item was consistently correct or incorrect in both the original and reliability transcriptions. Disagreement was confirmed if the transcription of the stimulus item was correct and incorrect in both the original and reliability transcriptions. The percentage of agreement between the original and reliability data was calculated using the following formula: [agreements/(agreements + disagreements)] × 100 = percentage of agreement (Tawney & Gast, 1984). Reliability percentages for each measurement condition were as follows: 1) word transcription without semantic context, 84%; 2) word transcription with semantic context, 90%; 3) sentence transcription without semantic context, 87%; and 4) sentence transcription with semantic context, 93%.

Measurement

Word and sentence intelligibility scores were obtained for each speaker for the four speaking conditions. Word and sentence intelligibility refer to the percentage of the total target words correctly transcribed. Individual word and sentence intelligibility scores obtained for all listeners in the four conditions were used for subsequent analyses.

RESULTS

A general overview of the results is seen in Table 2, which contains the mean intelligibility scores and standard deviations for each of the severity classifications and each of the measurement conditions.

To evaluate the interaction of semantic context, utterance length, and severity of the dysarthria, a three-way split plot ANOVA with a nested factor (Keppel, 1991) was run. The main effects of semantic context ($F = 91.91$, $p = .0007$) and severity of dysarthria ($F = 96.60$, $p = .0008$) were both significant, as was the interaction of semantic context and utterance length ($F = 33.94$, $p = .0043$) and utterance length and severity of the dysarthria ($F = 8.93$, $p = .0303$). The three-way interaction between utterance length, semantic context, and severity of the dysarthria was not

Table 2. Mean intelligibility scores and standard deviations

Severity level	Speaker number	WI score—no semantic context (%)	SD	WI score—with semantic context (%)	SD	SI score—no semantic context (%)	SD	SI score—with semantic context (%)	SD
Profound	1	0.33	1.15	30	7.33	0.30	1.15	8	8.00
	2	5.0	3.01	31	13.24	0.00	0.00	1	2.48
Severe	3	45.0	11.73	76	5.11	63.00	6.45	70	10.71
	4	40.0	9.02	88	7.32	77.00	12.31	84	9.94
Moderate	5	52.0	10.98	80	5.65	69.00	9.99	86	6.70
	6	54.0	10.84	93	7.45	82.00	10.01	98	3.11
Mild	7	72.0	7.03	96	3.41	98.00	2.67	98	3.61
	8	95.0	3.55	98	2.08	99.00	1.55	99	1.55

WI = Word intelligibility.
SI = Sentence intelligibility.

Table 3. Summary of the ANOVA results

Source of variation	Sum of squares	df	Mean square	F	Significance of F
Main effects					
Semantic context	30888.375	1	30888.4	91.91	.007
Utterance lengths	2109.375	1	2109.4	4.48	.1017
Severity	386777.125	3	128925.7	96.60	.0008
2-Way interaction					
Semantic context/ utterance length	11748.375	1	11748.4	33.94	.0043
Semantic context/ severity	4800.125	3	1600.0	4.75	.0832
Utterance length/severity	12605.125	3	4201.7	8.93	.0303
3-Way interaction					
Semantic context/ severity/utterance length	1241.458	3	413.8	1.20	.4179

significant ($F = 1.20$, $p = .4179$). Table 3 provides a summary of the findings from the ANOVA.

Because of the complexity of the nested factor in the ANOVA, follow-up t-tests were used to explore the significant interactions between utterance length and semantic context, as well as utterance length and severity of the dysarthria. Because of the large number of t-tests performed, the data were interpreted conservatively. Only those effects with a significance level of .01 or less were considered to be statistically significant. All the follow-up t-tests were significant at the t values, in addition to their associated significance levels, which are tabulated in Tables 4 and 5.

Table 4. Follow-up t-tests for the severity of the dysarthria and utterance length interaction

Severity	M	SD	SE	t value	df	2-Tail probability
Mild						
Word	90.17	6.85	1.39			
Sentence	98.58	1.99	.408	−6.61	23	.000
Moderate						
Word	69.58	7.41	1.51			
Sentence	83.83	8.82	1.80	−10.57	23	.000
Severe						
Word	62.41	5.82	1.15			
Sentence	73.33	10.39	2.12	−5.16	23	.000
Profound						
Word	17.17	5.81	1.19			
Sentence	2.88	8.42	.71	10.10	23	.000

Table 5. Follow-up *t*-tests for the semantic context and utterance length interaction

	M	SD	SE	*t* value	df	2-Tail probability
No semantic context						
Word	45.33	30.61	3.12	17.50	95	.000
Sentence	61.08	37.89	3.86	−9.70	95	.000
Semantic context						
Word	74.33	26.27	2.72			
Sentence	67.95	38.52	3.93	6.44	95	.000

DISCUSSION

This discussion highlights the effects of utterance length and semantic context on the speech intelligibility of speakers with flaccid dysarthria. The individual transcriptional intelligibility scores, obtained in each of the measurement conditions for each speaker, were averaged and the mean intelligibility scores for the speakers in each of the severity classifications were used to construct performance function curves (see Figures 1, 2, and 3). The initial single-word intelligibility measures were used to rank order the dysarthric speakers from profound to mildly impaired along the severity of dysarthria continuum. These curves illustrate the effects and nature of the interaction between utterance length, semantic context, and severity of the intelligibility disorder.

Utterance Length: Words versus Sentences

The results of this research study are consistent with previous research investigating the effects of utterance length on speech intelligibility (McGarr, 1981; 1983; Sitler et al., 1983; Yorkston & Beukelman, 1978). Intelligibility can be improved significantly in the presence of a distorted signal by increasing listener knowledge through increased utterance length. More specifically, there is a superiority of sentence over single-word intelligibility for the severe, moderate, and mild speaking groups. However, this trend was not evident for the profound group with single-word intelligibility significantly greater than sentence intelligibility (Figure 1).

Figure 1 also illustrates the interaction between utterance length and severity of the intelligibility impairment. Although post hoc testing revealed significant differences in intelligibility scores at all four levels of dysarthria severity, Table 4 shows that the magnitude of the differences varied as a function of severity, with the greatest improvements recorded for the group with severe dysarthria.

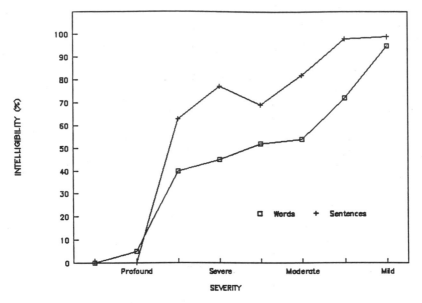

Figure 1. Performance function curves for words versus sentences.

The results of this study confirm previous research indicating that there is a point where the speech signal is so distorted that intelligibility cannot be influenced regardless of attempts to increase listener knowledge through increased utterance length. In fact, utterance length actually resulted in a decrease in the overall intelligibility scores for the speakers with profound dysarthria. For these profoundly impaired speakers, Yorkston and Beukelman (1978) inferred that sentence production was too demanding for the significantly disrupted respiratory, laryngeal, and articulatory systems of these individuals and therefore, absent of syntactic contextual cues. If this were solely the case, one might expect that single-word and sentence intelligibility would be roughly equivalent for these speakers. The fact that there was a significant difference between these two conditions suggests that there may be another contributing factor for the intelligibility decline.

It may be that sentence length signals produced by these profoundly impaired speakers are so distorted that syntactic contextual cues not only are absent but rather, the increased stimulus length provides the listener with information that detracts from the speech signal. Therefore, for profoundly impaired speakers, instead of the speech signal and listener knowledge serving complementary roles, as predicted by the mutuality model, they actually present conflicting roles, resulting in a decrease in successful communication.

Semantic Context

Table 5 reports the *t* values, in addition to their associated significance levels, for the comparisons of words and sentences with and without semantic context.

Words The effect of semantic context was powerful. The average percentage correct for the words in the no semantic context conditions was 45.33, and the average percentage correct for words in the context condition was 74.33. This difference was statistically significant ($t = 17.50, p = <.001$). Moreover, semantic context resulted in an increase in intelligibility scores for all severity groups. Figure 2 reflects this increase and illustrates the interaction between semantic context and severity of the intelligibility impairment. As with syntactic context, the greater improvement was noted for the severe group whose intelligibility scores increased 40.5%. These results are consistent with those reported by Hammen et al. (1991).

Sentences The results reported here are somewhat surprising. Providing semantic context during sentence intelligibility tasks resulted in an increase in intelligibility score for all speaking groups however, the effects were not nearly as great as those noted for single words (Figure 3).

The average percentage correct for the sentences in the no semantic context condition was 61.08, and the average percentage correct for sentences in the context condition was 67.95. Although this difference was

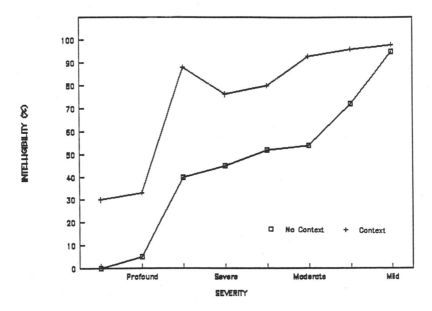

Figure 2. Performance function curves for words with and without semantic context.

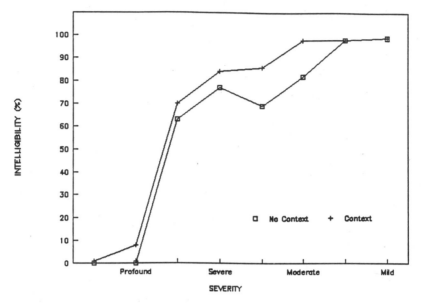

Figure 3. Performance function curves for sentences with and without semantic context.

statistically significant ($t = 3.96$, $p = <.001$), the functional importance could be questioned. Again, an interaction between semantic context and severity of the intelligibility impairment was evident. However, unlike the syntactic and single-word semantic context conditions, the greatest improvements were not noted for the severe group but rather for the moderate group. This group demonstrated a 16% increase in intelligibility scores in the semantic context condition.

These results are surprising in light of the powerful effect of semantic context with single words. Furthermore, the mutuality model implies that the cues provided to the listener as a result of increasing utterance length and semantic contextual cues would complement one another and act to increase speech intelligibility significantly. One explanation for these results is that the cues provided to the listener as a result of increasing utterance length may override the semantic contextual cues. Listeners may be more experienced at using cues provided secondary to increased utterance length in order to facilitate speech intelligibility. If put in a situation where listeners are provided with both, they may initially use the increased utterance length cues to aid intelligibility. As previously discussed, for at least the profound group, these increased utterance length cues may provide the listener with information that detracts from the speech signal. With a possible incorrect initial perception of the message established, the listener then utilizes the semantic contextual cue. If this cue is incongruent with the initial perception of the message, the listener may discard or ignore it. Therefore, sentence intelligibility will be roughly equivalent in the two conditions for the profound and severe groups.

CONCLUSIONS

The results of this study suggest that the speech intelligibility of speakers with flaccid dysarthria can be improved significantly, in the presence of a distorted signal, by increasing listener knowledge through increased utterance length and semantic context. Speech intelligibility tasks that take these factors into account may provide a more realistic measure of overall functional communication.

REFERENCES

Bigler, R.C. (1984). Speech recognition test development. In E. Elkins (Ed.), *ASHA Reports Number 14, Speech Recognition by The Hearing Impaired* (pp. 2–15). Rockville, MD: American Speech-Language-Hearing Association.

Darley, F.L., Aronson, A.E., & Brown, J.R. (1975). *Motor speech disorders.* Philadelphia: W.B. Saunders.

Hammen, V.L., Yorkston, K. M., & Dowden, P. (1991). Index of contextual intelligibility: Impact of semantic context in dysarthria. In C.A. Moore, K.M. Yorkston, & D.R. Beukelman (Eds.), *Dysarthria and apraxia of speech: Perspectives on management* (pp. 43–53). Baltimore: Paul H. Brookes Publishing Co.

Kalikow, D.N., Stevens, K.N., & Elliott, L.L. (1977). Development of a test of speech intelligibility in noise using sentence materials with controlled word predictability. *Journal of the Acoustical Society of America, 61,* 1339–1351.

Keppel, G. (1991). *Design and analysis: A researcher's handbook* (3rd ed.). Englewood Cliffs, NJ: Prentice Hall.

Lindblom, B. (1990). On the communication process: Speaker–listener interaction and the development of speech. *Augmentative and Alternative Communication, 6,* 220–230.

McGarr, N.S. (1981). The effect of context on the intelligibility of hearing and deaf children's speech. *Language and Speech, 24,* 255–264.

McGarr, N.S. (1983). The intelligibility of deaf speech to experienced and inexperienced listeners. *Journal of Speech and Hearing Research, 26,* 451–458.

Monsen, R.B. (1983). The oral speech intelligibility of hearing-impaired talkers. *Journal of Speech and Hearing Disorders, 48,* 286–296.

Sitler, R.W., Schiavetti, N., & Metz, D.E. (1983). Contextual effects in the measurement of hearing-impaired speakers' intelligibility. *Journal of Communication Disorders, 11,* 22–30.

Tawney, J.S., & Gast, D.L. (1984). *Single subject research in special education.* Columbus, OH: Bell and Howard.

Yorkston, K.M., & Beukelman, D.R. (1978). A comparison of techniques for measuring intelligibility of dysarthric speech. *Journal of Communication Disorders, 11,* 499–512.

Yorkston, K.M., & Beukelman, D.R. (1981). *Assessment of intelligibility of dysarthric speech.* Tigard, OR: C.C. Publications.

Appendix A

Stimulus Words

Risk
Spoon
Ox
Steam
Coin
Drug
Lap
Bone
Tanks
Gin
Oath
Den
Calf

Silk
Lanes
Pie
Mugs
Blush
Clock
Sword
Braids
Map
Crash
Pet
Wits

Stimulus Words and Semantic Contextual Cues

Words	Cues
Chest	Human body
Ditch	Digging
Swan	Birds
Joints	Arthritis
Pole	Flag
Clue	Guessing game
Cruise	Sailing
Bark	Dogs
Pork	Pigs
Tea	Drinks
Geese	Birds
Dent	Car accident
Sheets	Bedding
Coach	Team
Throat	Human body
Cap	Clothing
Wheat	Grain
Bread	Food
Logs	Fireplace
Roar	Lions
Strap	Seat belts
Firm	Mattress
Prize	Winning an award
Bomb	Explosion
Stripe	Zebra

Stimulus Sentences

Kill the bugs with this spray.
How much can I buy for a dime?
We shipped the furniture by truck.
My TV has a twelve-inch screen.
That accident gave me a scare.
The king wore a golden crown.
The girl swept the floor with a broom.
The nurse gave him first aid.
She faced them with a foolish grin.
Watermelons have lots of seeds.
Use this spray to kill the bugs.
The teacher sat on a sharp tack.
The sailor swabbed the deck.
He tossed the drowning man a rope.
The boy gave the football a kick.
The storm broke the sailboat's mast.
Mr. Brown carved the roast beef.
The glass had a chip on the rim.
Her cigarette had a long ash.
The soup was served in a bowl.
The lonely bird searched for its mate.
Please wipe your feet on the mat.
The pond was full of croaking frogs.
He hit me with a clenched fist.
A bicycle has two wheels.

Appendix D

Stimulus Sentences and Semantic Contextual Cues

Sentences	Cues
The baby slept in his crib.	Children
The watchdog gave a warning growl.	Protection
The natives built a wooden hut.	Island dwellers
Unlock the door and turn the knob.	Entering a house
Wipe your greasy hands on the rag.	Mechanics
The wedding banquet was a feast.	Celebration
Paul hit the water with a splash.	Swimming
The ducks swam around the pond.	Park
Bob stood with his hands on his hips.	Angry parent
The cigarette smoke filled his lungs.	Cancer
The cushion was filled with foam.	Upholstery
Ruth poured the water down the drain.	Cleaning dishes
This nozzle sprays a fine mist.	Washing a car
The sport shirt has short sleeves.	Clothing
She shortened the hem of her skirt.	Altering/sewing
The guests were welcomed by the host.	Dinner party
The ship's captain summoned his crew.	Sea travel
The flood took a heavy toll.	Natural disaster
The car drove off the steep cliff.	Automobile accident
The policemen captured the crook.	Robbery investigation
The door was opened just a crack.	Robbery investigation
The sand was heaped in a pile.	Beach
Household goods are moved in a van.	Moving
Follow this road around the bend.	Giving directions
The farmer baled the hay.	Chores

191

Comparisons of Fundamental Frequency Measures of Speakers with Dysarthria and Hyperfunctional Voice Disorders

Mark E. Hakel,
E. Charles Healey, and Marsha Sullivan

RECENT ADVANCES IN technology have led to the development of several microcomputer-based speech analysis systems, many of which are capable of measuring vocal fundamental frequency (Fo), a central component of voice analysis and prosodic characteristics of speech. Analysis of Fo has been developed for dedicated units or as a component of a larger speech analysis system hosted by a microcomputer. Fundamental frequency analysis functions developed for IBM-compatible computers are included in *CSpeech* (Milenkovic, 1990), and *MSL* (Software Research Corporation, 1985) systems. Fundamental frequency analysis functions for Apple computers are included in the *MacSpeech Lab II* (GW Instruments, Inc., 1988) and *CHIP* (Charlie Healey Interface Program) developed by Healey and Tice (1991).

Several years ago, Kay Elemetrics Corporation (1989) developed VISI-PITCH, a dedicated unit for pitch analysis. This system is available as a software package for the Apple IIe computers or IBM PC. Another dedicated unit for Fo analysis is the *PM Pitch Analyzer* (Voice Identification, Inc., 1981).

These systems have become popular in clinical, educational, and/or hospital settings because of their low cost and their increased user friendliness. Given this, Kerr, Healey, and Votipka (1990) conducted a systematic comparison of five popular Fo systems. They found that there was a high degree of consistency in the Fo values reported by *MSL* (Software, 1985), *MacSpeech Lab II* (GW, 1988), *VISI-PITCH* (Kay, 1984), *PM Pitch Analyzer* (Voice, 1981), and *CHIP* (Healey & Tice, 1991) for a group of adult female speakers with normal voices. Only small differences were noted between the Fo mean and standard deviations among these five systems when voice samples were taken from a sustained /a/ vowel and a sentence from the Rainbow Passage (Fairbanks, 1960). Kerr et al. (1990) concluded that it was possible to obtain a consistent measure of Fo from any of the five systems tested for adult females without voice disorders.

However, how these Fo systems compare when disordered voices are analyzed remains unknown. Read, Buder, and Kent (1992) suggested that many speech analysis systems would have difficulty analyzing pathological voices, caused by failure of the automatic Fo extraction algorithms.

This study examines the consistency of Fo values among the five Fo analysis systems studied by Kerr et al. (1990) when assessing disordered voices. Specifically, the Fo means and standard deviations of three groups of speakers with abnormal voice characteristics were compared. Comparisons were made among a group of speakers with hypokinetic dysarthria, a group of speakers with mixed dysarthrias, and a group with hyperfunctional voice disorders. Secondarily, we assessed any relationships between severity rating of voice disorders and consistency of Fo values among the five Fo analysis systems.

METHODS

Subjects

The group with hypokinetic dysarthria was comprised of six individuals (five males and one female) diagnosed with Parkinson's disease. The second group consisted of five speakers with dysarthria (four males and one female). One of the subjects demonstrated ataxic dysarthria, two showed flaccid dysarthric characteristics, and two were diagnosed with ataxic/spastic dysarthria. A third group of speakers was comprised of six adult females diagnosed with a hyperfunctional voice disorder. All of these subjects' voice disorders were caused by vocal abuse or misuse.

Each subject with dysarthria and a hyperfunctional voice disorder was diagnosed by an ASHA-certified speech-language pathologist. None was suffering from a cold, flu, a sore throat, or allergies at the time of the testing. All were medically stable.

Description of Fo Analysis Systems

The five dedicated hardware and software systems included: 1) *CHIP* (Healey & Tice, 1991), an Apple IIe/gs software system; 2) *MSL* (Software, 1985), an IBM software system; 3) *MacSpeech Lab II*, Version 1.4, a Macintosh software system (GW, 1988); 4) *PM Pitch Analyzer* (201 Program), a dedicated hardware system (Voice, 1981); and 5) the *VISI-PITCH* (Model #6095), an Apple IIe software system (Kay, 1984). These systems were chosen because of their popularity among and availability to clinicians and researchers. Hardware requirements and features of each Fo analysis system are shown in Table 1. For an in-depth description of features of *MSL* and *MacSpeech II*, in addition to other acoustic systems, see Read, Buder, and Kent (1990, 1992).

Procedures

Voice samples were obtained during a portion of a subject's treatment or diagnostic session. Each subject was recorded individually in a quiet room. An electret-condenser microphone was positioned 15 cm from the subject's lips and connected to a high-quality tape-recorder (Marantz # PMD 420). Once seated and properly positioned, each subject was instructed to read the first paragraph of the Rainbow Passage (Fairbanks, 1960) once.

Data Analysis

From each subject's tape-recorded sample, the second sentence—*The rainbow is a division of white light into many beautiful colors.*—was used to obtain the Fo measures. This sentence was chosen because Horii (1975) found that it yielded Fo values that closely matched the Fo value for the entire paragraph. Prior to Fo analysis, each subject's recording was filtered at 4kHz in order to eliminate high-frequency noise components on the tape that might have interfered with the Fo analysis. Each filtered recording was then played into each of the five Fo analysis systems.

Because each speech analysis system calculates Fo differently, the number of data points obtained from each system also varied. Thus, in order to compare the Fo values obtained from the five systems, an attempt was made to keep the quantity of data for analysis relatively similar. For the *MSL* (Software, 1985), *MacSpeech* (GW, 1988), and *CHIP* (Healey & Tice, 1991) systems, an Fo value was chosen at approximately every 50 ms interval from the beginning to the end of all periodic phonation segments within the sample. Mean and standard deviation values were calculated from the Fo values at these 50 ms intervals for each subject. All 50 ms

Table 1. Features and hardware requirements of each Fo analysis system

Equipment	CHIP	MSL (version 3.0)	MacSpeech Lab II (version 1.4)	VISI-PITCH (#6095)	PM/Pitch Analyzer (201 Program)
Computer	Apple IIe/gs	PC/AT	Macintosh II	Apple IIe	Dedicated unit
A/D, D/A board(s)	Required	Included	Included	Included	Included
Input/output filters	Required	Included	Included	Included	Included
Sampling rate	10 or 20 kHz	10 or 20 kHz	10, 20, 40, 80 kHz	100 kHz	Unknown
Waveform display	Yes	Yes	Yes	No	No
Statistical data	M, SD perturbation	None	None	M, perturbation max Fo/min Fo	M, SD
Method of determining Fo	Period value between amplitude peaks	Period value between amplitude peaks	Autocorrelation	Zero crossing (Hysteresus)	Zero crossing

segments were averaged to derive a grand Fo mean and standard deviation value. This averaging procedure was less time consuming and more practical than using all the data. Weinberg and Bennett (1972) confirmed that an averaging procedure such as that used in the present study yields comparable mean Fo values obtained from wave-by-wave analysis.

In contrast to the above systems, the *VISI-PITCH* (Kay, 1984) and *PM Pitch Analyzer* (Voice, 1981) provide a screen display that permits the user to place the cursors at the beginning and end of the speech signal. The average Fo is calculated between the cursors and displayed on the screen. In the present study, the left cursor was placed at the beginning of the signal and the right cursor was moved in approximately 70 msec steps through the entire waveform. A new Fo mean value was displayed at each new cursor location. Each Fo value displayed on the screen was then recorded on a sheet of paper and an Fo mean and standard deviation were derived for each subject.

Severity Ratings

A group of seven graduate students who had recently completed a Master's degree-level voice course rated the hyperfunctional voices. The speakers with dysarthria were rated by five ASHA-certified speech-language pathologists working in an acute rehabilitation facility where they had extensive clinical experience with patients with dysarthria. Each group was instructed to rate the parameter of hoarseness on a 7-point scale with 1 representing the absence of hoarseness and 7 representing severe or extreme hoarseness. The ratings for each voice were totaled and then averaged. Voices rated on an average of 2–3 were classified as mild; 4–5 as moderate; and 6–7 as severe. The judges were instructed to ignore all other speech parameters when rating the voice samples. Based on the judgments made, 12 voices were judged as mildly hoarse, four were moderately hoarse, and one was severely hoarse. All ratings of severity were made without regard to speaker classification.

RESULTS

Speakers with Hypokinetic Dysarthria

Table 2 shows the comparisons of Fo mean and standard deviation differences for all possible pairs of Fo analysis systems. Fo mean differences ranged from 4.7–13.7 Hz with a mean of 9.3 Hz. The smallest difference was associated with the Fo values between *MacSpeech* (GW, 1988) and *PM Pitch Analyzer* (Voice, 1981). The largest difference in Fo occurred between the values obtained for *MSL* (Software, 1985) and *CHIP* (Healey, & Tice, 1991).

Table 2. Comparison of Fo mean and standard deviation differences (in Hz) between pairs of Fo analysis systems for speakers with hypokinetic dysarthria

Systems	Hypokinetic dysarthria	
	Fo M difference	Fo SD difference
MSL vs. MAC	13.5	10.2
MSL vs. PM	11.5	10.3
MSL vs. CHIP	13.7	7.8
MSL vs. VISI	8.3	6.7
MAC vs. PM	4.7	4.2
MAC vs. CHIP	9.5	6.7
MAC vs. VISI	8.2	8.4
PM vs. CHIP	8.8	4.6
PM vs. VISI	5.5	5.6
CHIP vs. VISI	9.7	7.3

As seen in Table 2, all 10 comparisons were within 5 Hz of the mean Fo difference. However, the three highest Fo mean differences were associated with systems compared to *MSL* (Software, 1985).

The Fo standard deviation differences shown in Table 2 (i.e., variability in Fo) ranged from 4.2 Hz to 10.3 Hz, with an average difference of 7.2 Hz. The smallest amount of variability was associated with the measures from *MacSpeech* (GW, 1988) and *PM Pitch Analyzer* (Voice, 1981). The largest difference occurred between *MSL* Software, 1985) and *PM Pitch Analyzer* (Voice, 1981).

Speakers with Mixed Dysarthria

Comparisons of Fo values from all the possible pairs of the five Fo analysis systems for the group with mixed dysarthria are shown in Table 3. The average Fo difference between any two systems was 8.5 Hz, which was

Table 3. Comparison of Fo mean and standard deviation differences (in Hz) between pairs of Fo analysis systems for a group of speakers with mixed dysarthria

Systems	Mixed dysarthria	
	Fo M difference	Fo SD difference
MSL vs. MAC	5.0	5.2
MSL vs. PM	10.4	6.7
MSL vs. CHIP	12.2	10.8
MSL vs. VISI	11.8	6.3
MAC vs. PM	7.8	7.0
MAC vs. CHIP	12.4	13.1
MAC vs. VISI	9.6	8.0
PM vs. CHIP	7.1	5.8
PM vs. VISI	3.0	2.6
CHIP vs. VISI	5.6	4.5

similar to the Fo difference for the hypokinetic voice comparisons. Fo mean differences ranged from 3 Hz–12.4 Hz. A 3 Hz difference occurred between the *PM Pitch Analyzer* (Voice, 1981) and *VISI-PITCH* (Kay, 1984) and a 12.4 Hz difference was found between *MacSpeech* (GW, 1988) and *CHIP* (Healey & Tice, 1991). It should also be noted that three of the four largest Fo mean differences were associated with systems paired with *MSL* (Software, 1985).

The average Fo standard deviation difference was 7 Hz, with a range of 2.6 Hz to 13.1 Hz. The smallest difference was found for the measures between the *PM Pitch Analyzer* (Voice, 1981) and *VISI-PITCH* (Kay, 1984). The largest difference in Fo variability was between *MacSpeech* (GW, 1988) and *CHIP* (Healey & Tice, 1991) analysis systems.

Speakers with Hyperfunctional Voice Disorder

The hyperfunctional voice data in Table 4 show larger Fo mean differences among the systems than for the speaker groups with hypokinetic and mixed dysarthrias.

From the data in Table 4, the average Fo mean difference was 15.2 Hz, ranging from 8.3 Hz to 23 Hz when all possible pairs of Fo systems were compared. A 8.3 Hz difference was found between *MacSpeech* (GW, 1981) and *PM Pitch Analyzer* (Voice, 1985), whereas a 23 Hz difference was found between *MSL* (Software, 1985) and *CHIP* (Healey & Tice, 1991). As seen with the other two speaker groups, three of the four largest Fo mean differences for the speakers with hyperfunction were associated with *MSL* (Software, 1985).

Average Fo standard deviation difference fluctuated from 7.9 Hz to 31.8 Hz, with a mean Fo variability of 14 Hz. A 7.9 Hz difference occurred between *MSL* (Software, 1985) and *VISI-PITCH* (Kay, 1984) as

Table 4. Comparison of Fo mean and standard deviation differences (in Hz) between pairs of Fo analysis systems for speakers with hyperfunctional voice disorders

Systems	Speakers with hyperfunctional voice disorders	
	Fo M difference	Fo SD difference
MSL vs. MAC	15.8	11.0
MSL vs. PM	16.5	8.2
MSL vs. CHIP	23.0	19.9
MSL vs. VISI	11.8	7.9
MAC vs. PM	8.3	7.9
MAC vs. CHIP	15.2	10.5
MAC vs. VISI	14.7	21.3
PM vs. CHIP	11.8	9.2
PM vs. VISI	13.7	20.5
CHIP vs. VISI	21.2	31.8

well as *MacSpeech* (GW, 1981) and *PM Pitch Analyzer* (Voice, 1981). A 31.8 Hz difference was found between *CHIP* (Healey & Tice, 1991) and *VISI-PITCH* (Kay, 1984).

Differences According to Severity

Fo mean differences according to severity are shown in Table 5. The data in this table show that the Fo mean difference for mild voices ranged from 3.9 to 14.4 Hz, with an average difference of 8.8 Hz. For moderately hoarse voices, the Fo mean difference ranged from 2.8 Hz to 18.3 Hz with an average of a 10.6 Hz difference. For one subject with severe hoarseness, the range of Fo difference was 2 Hz to 83 Hz, with an average difference of 39.6 Hz.

Average standard deviation differences between the five analysis systems for each severity category are shown in Table 6. The differences in the group with mild hoarseness ranged from 5.3 Hz to 10.8 Hz with a mean difference of 8.3 Hz. The group with moderately hoarse voices showed a range of differences from 2.5 Hz to 47.7 Hz with an average difference of 13.5 Hz. The subject rated as severely hoarse exhibited a range of standard deviation differences from 1 Hz to 23 Hz with an average of 11.2 Hz difference.

DISCUSSION

This study revealed that the five speech analysis systems used in this experiment produced more consistent Fo values for the subjects with dysarthria than for the speakers with hyperfunction. In fact, the mean Fo differences among the five systems for the speakers with dysarthria was similar to the mean Fo difference reported by Kerr et al. (1990) for a group

Table 5. Comparison of Fo mean differences between pairs of Fo analysis systems by severity rating

	Severity		
Systems	Mild (*n* = 12)	Moderate (*n* = 4)	Severe (*n* = 1)
MSL vs. MAC	7.5	15.2	32
MSL vs. PM	9.8	18.3	30
MSL vs. CHIP	12.1	18.3	58
MSL vs. VISI	8.8	12.3	25
MAC vs. PM	6.9	5.5	2
MAC vs. CHIP	14.4	2.8	26
MAC vs. VISI	8.2	10.5	57
PM vs. CHIP	8.7	7.8	28
PM vs. VISI	3.9	7.0	55
CHIP vs. VISI	8.1	8.3	83

Table 6. Comparison of Fo standard deviation differences between pairs of Fo analysis systems by severity rating

Systems	Severity		
	Mild (n = 12)	Moderate (n = 4)	Severe (n = 1)
MSL vs. MAC	5.3	10.2	10
MSL vs. PM	7.3	16.2	1
MSL vs. CHIP	10.2	47.7	13
MSL vs. VISI	7.3	6.5	10
MAC vs. PM	9.3	8.0	9
MAC vs. CHIP	10.5	10.5	3
MAC vs. VISI	8.2	2.5	20
PM vs. CHIP	10.8	15.5	12
PM vs. VISI	5.3	8.0	11
CHIP vs. VISI	8.3	10.0	23

of nondisabled female voices. Data from these voices showed a mean Fo difference of approximately 9 Hz, whereas the mean Fo differences for the groups with hypokinetic and mixed dysarthrias were 9 Hz and 8.5 Hz, respectively. The comparable mean Fo differences between the dysarthric and nondisabled voices suggest that there were minimal waveform irregularities associated with the hypokinetic and mixed dysarthric voices. As a result, all five speech analysis systems seem capable of determining Fo mean and standard deviation values from these voices.

Voices rated as either mild or moderately hoarse also showed similar Fo mean differences among the five systems. The average Fo mean difference for the voices with mild hoarseness was approximately 9 Hz and about 10.5 Hz for voices rated moderately hoarse. These data show that even moderate hoarseness, which would contain a reasonable degree of waveform aperiodicity, does not adversely affect the analysis capabilities of any one of the five speech systems. This finding is important because many dysarthric voices and most hyperfunctional voices will possess mild to moderate hoarseness (Aronson, 1985; Case, 1991).

In contrast to the findings above, it should be noted that the hyperfunctional voice samples showed a higher Fo mean difference than the dysarthric voices and those voices rated mildly to moderately hoarse. The higher mean Fo difference for the speakers with hyperfunctional voices probably was attributable to one subject with severe vocal hoarseness. This subject had large mean Fo differences among the five speech systems. These large values served to inflate the group mean Fo difference. One would expect that a voice judged to be severely dysphonic would contain more waveform aperiodicity than a voice judged to be mildly dysphonic. Thus, with the exception of the severely hyperfunctional voice, there does not seem to be a large difference in Fo means from one speech analysis system to another for the group of mildly and moderately hyperfunctional voice disordered speakers.

The clinician must decide whether or not the differences in mean Fo among the systems are acceptable for treatment or research purposes. The data from the present study can serve as a guide for which system(s) to use for Fo analysis. It is encouraging that there are small differences in Fo measures among the systems for mildly and moderately hoarse dysarthric and hyperfunctional voices. It seems that dedicated systems, such as the *PM Pitch Analyzer* (Voice, 1981) and *VISI-PITCH* (Kay, 1984), produced Fo measurements for the mildly to moderately dysarthric and hyperfunctional voices that were similar to the microcomputer-based systems.

However, the clinician may want to determine a client's Fo with more than one system, especially if the degree of hoarseness is perceived as severe. These voices contain excessive amounts of cycle-to-cycle variability within the signal and automated Fo analysis systems have difficulty extracting Fo consistently. For these aperiodic voices, a system such as *CHIP* (Healey & Tice, 1991) may be required to allow the clinician to mark manually the signal to be analyzed. The *VISI-PITCH* (Kay, 1984) and *PM Pitch Analyzer* (Voice, 1981) do not allow the user to view the recorded and analyzed waveform. In contrast, systems such as *CHIP* (Healey & Tice, 1991), *MSL* (Software, 1985), and *MacSpeech Lab* (GW, 1988) can display a waveform and allow the user to measure Fo for small segments within the speech signal. Although the analysis time is longer with these three systems than with dedicated Fo units, the user can inspect the Fo data and choose representative Fo values. For this reason, researchers may prefer these types of Fo extraction systems.

In conclusion, it seems that any of the five systems would provide adequate Fo information for the dysarthric and mildly to moderately hyperfunctional voices. However, there is an obvious need to expand the size of the study to evaluate severe hoarseness with dysarthric and hyperfunctional voices. The findings from this study support Read et al.'s (1992) suggestion that new and alternative means of representing the speech signal need to be developed. Perhaps a system that would allow the user to set analysis parameters might limit signal artifact or noise from being introduced into the Fo analysis process.

REFERENCES

Aronson, A.E. (1985). *Clinical voice disorders: An interdisciplinary approach*. New York: Thieme Medical Publishers, Inc.

Case, J.L. (1991). *Clinical management of voice disorders*. Austin, TX: PRO-ED.

Fairbanks, F. (1960). *Voice and articulation drillbook*. New York: Harper & Row.

GW Instruments, Inc. (1988). *MacSpeech Lab II* [Computer program]. 35 Medford Street, Somerville, MA 02143.

Healey, E.C., & Tice, R. (1991). A fundamental frequency and intensity analysis program for the Apple IIe/gs. *Journal for Computer Users in Speech and Hearing*, 7, 28–34.

Horii, Y. (1975). Some statistical characteristics of voice fundamental frequency. *Journal of Speech and Hearing Research*, 18, 192–201.

Kay Elemetrics Corporation. (1984). *VISI-PITCH* [Computer program]. 3939 Quadra Street, Victoria, BC, V8X 1J5, Canada.

Kerr, M., Healey, E.C., & Votipka, J. (1990). *Comparison of fundamental frequency measures across three microcomputer systems*. Paper presented at American Speech-Language-Hearing Association, Seattle, WA.

Milenkovic, P. (1990). *CSpeech* [Computer program]. Department of Electrical and Computer Engineering, University of Wisconsin-Madison, 1415 Johnson Drive, Madison, WI 53706.

Read C., Buder, E., & Kent, R. (1990). Speech analysis systems: A survey. *Journal of Speech and Hearing Research*, 33, 363–374.

Read, C., Buder, E., & Kent, R. (1992). Speech analysis systems: An evaluation. *Journal of Speech and Hearing Research*, 35, 314–332.

Software Research Corporation. (1985). *MSL* [Computer program]. 3939 Quadra Street, Victoria, BC, V8X 1J5, Canada.

Voice Identification, Inc. (1981). *PM Pitch Analyzer* [Computer program]. P.O. Box 714, Somerville, NJ 08876.

Weinberg, B., & Bennett, S. (1972). A comparison of the fundamental frequency characteristics of esophageal speech measured on a wave-by-wave and averaging basis. *Journal of Speech and Hearing Research*, 15, 351–355.

SECTION IV

APPROACHES
TO TREATMENT

Chapter 15

CPAP Therapy for Treating Hypernasality Following Closed Head Injury

David P. Kuehn and Jayne M. Wachtel

CONTINUOUS POSITIVE AIRWAY pressure, commonly called CPAP, has been used routinely to treat patients with obstructive sleep apnea (Schmidt-Nowara, 1984). An air pressure-flow device is used to deliver air to the nasal cavities via a hose and nasal mask assembly. The person with apnea wears the mask during sleep. The positive air pressure delivered to the nasal cavities prevents collapse of the upper airway, thus keeping the airway patent and allowing the person to breathe while sleeping.

The positive air pressure provides a resistance against which the muscles of velopharyngeal closure must work. Theoretically, this activity could be used in a resistance exercise paradigm to strengthen the muscles of velopharyngeal closure, thereby reducing hypernasality. Preliminary work with such a therapeutic approach in treating speakers with hypernasality following closed head injury is described in this chapter.

CPAP THERAPY PROCEDURE

The therapy technique has been described in detail elsewhere (Kuehn, 1991) and only the essentials are discussed here. We have been using

This work was supported by Grant No. 1 R03 DC01015-01 from the National Institute on Deafness and Other Communication Disorders.
This work is in the public domain.

equipment supplied by Respironics Inc., Murrysville, Pennsylvania. The most recent model is *REMstar*.

Treatment is a home therapy program. Typically, the total length of therapy is 8 weeks, with six sessions per week. Daily sessions vary from 10 minutes per session the first week to 24 minutes per session the eighth week. Table 1 shows the schedule and the pressures used for each session. It can be seen that the lowest pressure setting is 4.0 cm H_2O and the highest is 8.5 cm H_2O. The pressures gradually increase over the course of therapy. The pattern is obvious in Table 1.

At the beginning of a session, the subject places the mask over the nose, ensuring an airtight seal around the nose, but leaving the lips unencumbered. The pressure for the session is then adjusted using a set screw on the CPAP machine. Pressure is calibrated using a U-tube water manometer available with the CPAP machine.

Speech drill work consists of repetition of single-word utterances of the form VNCV in which V = any vowel, N = any nasal consonant, and C = any "pressure" consonant (stop, fricative, affricate), provided that the sequence is phonologically permissible. Emphatic stress is placed on the second syllable. The rationale for the particular phonemic sequence is that the nasal consonant induces a lowered velar position and the pressure consonant initiating the stressed syllable enhances the likelihood of a rigorous velar elevation. Such activity in the presence of heightened nasal air pressure theoretically takes advantage of the resistance exercise situation.

Fifty VNCV words are produced per list, followed by six short sentences. This pattern is repeated using additional words and sentences until the end of the session. Sentences are used in addition to nonsense words because they are closer to natural speech, thus helping to generalize the higher effort level to conversational speech. The sentences consist of three sentences with and three without nasal consonants. Older subjects read these materials and younger subjects, or those who need special assistance, are prompted by a care provider.

CASE STUDIES

Subject 1, J.S.

Subject 1 was in an accident at 18 years of age when he was thrown through the windshield of a car, sustaining a closed head injury. On admission to the trauma center, he was deeply comatose and reacted with decerebrate movements of the limbs to noxious stimulation.

Computerized tomography (CT) on admission showed questionable accumulation of blood in the right hemisphere. A follow-up CT scan

Table 1. Therapy schedule: pressure settings and time per session

Week	Monday CPAP[a]	Monday Time[b]	Tuesday CPAP	Tuesday Time	Wednesday CPAP	Wednesday Time	Thursday CPAP	Thursday Time	Friday CPAP	Friday Time	Saturday CPAP	Saturday Time
1	4.0	10	4.5	10	5.0	10	4.0	10	4.5	10	4.5	10
2	4.5	12	5.0	12	5.5	12	4.5	12	5.0	12	5.0	12
3	5.0	14	5.5	14	6.0	14	5.0	14	5.5	14	5.5	14
4	5.5	16	6.0	16	6.5	16	5.5	16	6.0	16	6.0	16
5	6.0	18	6.5	18	7.0	18	6.0	18	6.5	18	6.5	18
6	6.5	20	7.0	20	7.5	20	6.5	20	7.0	20	7.0	20
7	7.0	22	7.5	22	8.0	22	7.0	22	7.5	22	7.5	22
8	7.5	24	8.0	24	8.5	24	7.5	24	8.0	24	8.0	24

[a]Pressure in cm H_2O.
[b]Minutes per session.

week later showed a 5-millimeter left subdural hematoma. A subsequent CT scan showed improvement, with minimal subdural fluid collection in the left hemisphere.

During the subject's hospitalization in an acute care facility, he required tracheostomy and gastrostomy tubes. He had focal seizures and was treated with Dilantin. The subject was nonverbal and agitated.

After 4 weeks, the subject was transferred to an inpatient rehabilitation center, where he received 10 weeks of intensive speech, occupational, and physical therapy. During this time, his gastrostomy and tracheostomy tubes were removed. The subject slowly began to verbalize and his level of awareness improved. His speech was described as moderately dysarthric.

Following inpatient rehabilitation, the subject received outpatient speech therapy four times per week for 3 months, and then two times per week for 4 months. Speech therapy during this period focused on improving his articulation skills. His resonance was described as hypernasal and his speech contained nasal emissions of air.

Because of his continued hypernasality the subject was seen by a cleft palate team approximately 1 1/2 years after his closed head injury. A lateral cephalometric study revealed minimal soft palate movement with good palatal length. A palatal lift prosthesis was recommended.

The lift was worn by the subject. Decreased hypernasality was reported with the lift in place. A lateral cephalometric study with the lift in place revealed soft palate movement with contact against the posterior pharyngeal wall while the subject sustained the /s/ sound. However, the subject was dissatisfied with the lift. He reported that it was uncomfortable and he did not feel that he was making significant progress with the prosthesis. Therefore, CPAP therapy was initiated.

At the beginning of CPAP therapy, the subject was evaluated by the first author as exhibiting a #4 severity rating on a 7-point scale, with #1 being normal and #7 being the most extreme hypernasality. Significant progress was made after 2 months of home therapy. The subject was highly motivated to continue his speech improvement; therefore, he continued for an additional month of home therapy, making a total of 3 months. Little improvement was detected at the 3 month return visit compared to 2 months, and CPAP therapy was terminated at that time.

The subject continued to exhibit dysarthria. However, with regard to resonance balance, he reduced hypernasality from a #4 to a #2 rating, with most improvement occurring within the first 4 weeks of therapy. He maintained reduced hypernasality and was rated at #2 1-year post CPAP therapy.

Subject 2, K.L.

Subject 2 was 16 years of age when his car hit a truck head on. He was ejected from the car and sustained a closed head injury. On admission to the emergency room, he was comatose and was moving his left upper extremity with some extensor posturing. A CT scan of the head revealed diffuse cerebral edema.

He was transferred to an acute care facility for four weeks where he received tracheostomy and gastrostomy tubes. He was then transferred to a rehabilitation center where he received approximately four months of intensive speech, occupational, and physical therapy. On discharge from the rehabilitation center, his speech was described as moderately dysarthric with hypernasality.

The subject received daily outpatient rehabilitation services, including speech therapy, for 6 months following his discharge. Speech therapy focused on improving his breath support, rate of speech, and articulation. Hypernasality continued to be a problem. He was approximately 70% intelligible during production of multisyllabic words.

Approximately 1 year following his accident, he was seen by a cleft palate team to evaluate his hypernasality. A nasendoscopic examination was performed. Inconsistent palatal movement was reported. Frontal and lateral views of the velopharyngeal region were obtained using videofluoroscopy. The frontal view revealed lateral pharyngeal wall movement that was inconsistent. The movement appeared sluggish initially, but later improved. The lateral view showed inconsistent palatal elevation. At some times, normal palatal elevation was observed. At other times, palatal elevation was found to be only fair with no contact against the posterior pharyngeal wall. Occasional air escape with overall weak phonation was reported. Because of these findings, a palatal lift was recommended.

The subject wore the palatal lift, but continued to experience hypernasality. A second videofluoroscopy was obtained with the palatal lift in place. It was observed that the lift restricted palatal movement and his speech seemed improved with the lift removed. CPAP therapy was recommended at this point.

Subject K.L.'s hypernasality was more severe than that of Subject J.S. at the beginning of therapy, about a #6 on the 7-point scale. K.L.'s course of therapy was complicated by his allergies. The heightened nasal air pressure from the CPAP machine increased the discomfort caused by his allergies and subject K.L. discontinued therapy for several days during the home treatment regimen. Nevertheless, both K.L. and his parents were motivated to continue therapy and he, as did subject J.S., continued for an additional month of home therapy, for a total of 3 months. K.L.'s father, in particular, was very pleased with K.L.'s progress and indicated that K.L.'s articulation, as well as his nasal resonance balance, had improved.

DISCUSSION

Theoretically, it seems that individuals with neurologic impairment related to closed head injury or other causes might benefit from CPAP therapy to reduce hypernasality. We are encouraged by the preliminary results. If effective, CPAP therapy has several advantages over traditional treatment using palatal lift prostheses, including: 1) increased subject comfort, 2) greater convenience, and 3) more active subject and care provider participation. All three of these were evident in the subjects of this report.

The third advantage listed above is particularly noteworthy. It seems that following closed head injury, individuals are very anxious to be involved in their own rehabilitation, especially with regard to speech. From the subject's perspective, and that of his or her caregiver, palatal lift management is a passive treatment approach. In contrast, CPAP therapy allows individuals to be very actively involved in their own management. Moreover, care providers also can be involved, as was the case with K.L.'s father, who was an extremely active participant.

Most of our experience with CPAP therapy involves subjects with hypernasality but without obvious neurologic involvement, such as individuals with cleft palate. We are studying a sample of the population with cleft palate to determine if CPAP therapy is effective in treating that group. However, we feel that treating patients with neurologic impairment using CPAP also has merit and we intend to explore that application for future subjects.

REFERENCES

Kuehn, D.P. (1991). New therapy for treating hypernasal speech using continuous positive airway pressure (CPAP). *Plastic and Reconstructive Surgery, 88,* 959–966.
Schmidt-Nowara, W.W. (1984). Continuous positive airway pressure for long-term treatment of sleep apnea. *American Journal of Diseases of Children, 138,* 82–92.

Chapter 16

Accelerating Speech in a Case of Hypokinetic Dysarthria
Descriptions and Treatment

Scott G. Adams

AKINETIC RIGID SYNDROMES, such as Parkinson's disease and progressive supranuclear palsy (PSP) typically are characterized by bradykinesia, that is, an abnormal slowing of movement. However, a certain proportion of patients with akinetic rigid syndromes exhibit a rapid and accelerating movement pattern. When this rapid movement affects the speech system, the result is referred to as *accelerating speech*. Darley, Aronson, and Brown (1975) indicated that four of 32, or 13%, of their patients with hypokinetic dysarthria demonstrated accelerating speech. They also observed that this very rapid pattern of speech production can become reduced to an unintelligible murmur, particularly toward the end of sentences (Darley et al., 1975). Unfortunately, few studies have attempted to determine the specific phonetic, acoustic, and physiologic parameters that may contribute to the intelligibility deficit associated with accelerating speech.

Most of the limited evidence available on accelerated speech and its effects on intelligibility are from a small number of treatment studies examining the effects of delayed auditory feedback (DAF) on accelerating parkinsonian speech. Auditory feedback delays, in the range of 50–150 msec, have been shown to produce a significant reduction in the speaking

This research was supported in part by a grant from the American Speech-Language-Hearing Association Foundation.

213

rate of individuals with accelerating dysarthria (Downie, Low, & Lindsay, 1981; Hanson & Metter, 1981; Hanson & Metter, 1983; Yorkston, Beukelman, & Bell, 1988). This reduction is reported to be associated with a marked improvement in intelligibility measures. Unfortunately, the measures of intelligibility used in these studies were restricted to clinical impressions (Downie et al., 1981), simple rating scales (Hanson & Metter, 1983), or global measures of severity (Yorkston et al., 1988).

For example, Hanson and Metter (1983) used a 7-point, equal appearing interval scale to rate the intelligibility of two Parkinson's patients with rapid speech. They reported more than a 3-point improvement in intelligibility for one patient when delayed auditory feedback was introduced. Similarly, Yorkston et al. (1988) used their intelligibility test and reported that the intelligibility of one Parkinson rapid speaker changed from a baseline score of 67% to a score of 97% when delayed auditory feedback was used.

Although these reports clearly indicate the effectiveness of delayed auditory feedback for the treatment of intelligibility deficits in accelerated speech, they do not provide information about the specific phonetic, acoustic, and kinematic parameters that were responsible for these changes in intelligibility. Such information could give us a better understanding of the nature of accelerated speech in hypokinetic dysarthria and also provide a better explanation for the intelligibility changes that occur as a result of delayed auditory feedback.

The present study provides detailed phonetic, acoustic, and kinematic descriptions of the intelligibility deficit seen in one speaker with hypokinetic dysarthria who presented with accelerated speech. This study also describes some of the changes in speech production associated with the patient's use of delayed auditory feedback.

METHODS

Subject

The patient was a 78-year-old male with a 2- to 3-year history of an akinetic-rigid syndrome, suspected to be progressive, supranuclear palsy. He demonstrated a prominent gait disturbance, significant postural instability, some axial rigidity, no limb rigidity, no tremor, and a slight disturbance in vertical eye movements. He had not been responsive to levodopa therapy and his magnetic resonance imaging (MRI) scan was normal. The patient exhibited marked acceleration of movement during repetitive limb tests, such as finger tapping and foot tapping, and his writing was micrographic.

The patient's speech disturbance was one of his major complaints. His speech was characterized by a rapid and accelerating pattern. Conversational speaking rate, measured after the interphrase pauses were removed, was 375 words per minute. Intelligibility was judged to be markedly reduced during conversation. An intelligibility score of 54% was obtained on the sentence version of the Computerized Assessment of Intelligibility of Dysarthric Speech (CAIDS) (Yorkston, Beukelman, & Traynor, 1984). The patient also had slightly reduced voice intensity and poor voice quality, perceived as both harsh and breathy.

Procedures

Perceptual/Phonetic Data Analysis The patient was administered a modified version of the phonetic intelligibility test (PIT) developed by Kent, Weismer, Kent, and Rosenbek (1989) for the assessment of speakers with dysarthria. For the present study, this single-word test was modified by including a task that required the patient to produce target words in repeated carrier phrases. Thus, the test's original 70 words were produced both in isolation and in the carrier phrase, "I'll say _____ again," which the patient repeated three times in succession. For example, a card with the test word "bad" would be presented and the patient would be required to say, "Bad [pause]. I'll say bad again. I'll say bad again. I'll say bad again." The addition of a repeated carrier phrase allowed for a more complete evaluation of the intelligibility deficit associated with an accelerating pattern of speech.

The patient first produced the items from this modified PIT using normal auditory feedback, and then using delayed auditory feedback. A portable DAF unit (Phone Ear PM505) was used to produce a constant auditory delay interval of 80 msec. Throughout the testing procedures, an audio recording of the patient's speech was made using a head-mounted microphone (TOA-HY3) and tape recorder (TASCAM 112R). The patient was seated in a sound-treated booth (Eckel 66S) during all testing.

The audio recordings were low-pass filtered (10 kHz) and digitized (20 kHz) using a personal computer and CSpeech software (Milenkovic, 1990). The editing features of CSpeech were used to segment the test words and carrier phrases. These test words and carrier phrases were then randomly presented to three speech-language pathologists for scoring. The scoring procedure required the listeners to select the correct target word from a list of four possible choices. For example, the listener might be presented with the patient's production of the word "bad" and would be required to select from among the choices "bad," "bed," "bat," and "pad." Each of the alternate choices differed from the target word by a single phonetic feature. The listeners' incorrect choices on the test words were used to construct a phonetic error profile of the patient's speech. For a more detailed description of these phonetic contrasts and the construction of the phonetic error profile the reader is referred to Kent et al. (1989).

Acoustic Analysis   The patient's digitized utterances were analyzed using amplitude-time waveforms and spectrographic displays produced by CSpeech. The duration of each utterance was determined by measuring the period between the first and last glottal pulse on the amplitude-time waveform. Spectrographic displays (0–5 kHz) were used to make a variety of observations about the acoustic parameters associated with this patient's accelerating pattern of speech production.

Kinematic Analysis   Kinematic data were obtained using the head-mounted lip/jaw movement transduction system, previously described by Barlow, Cole, and Abbs (1983). Specifically, this system was used to record the inferior–superior movements of points on the upper lip, lower lip, and jaw during the various speech tasks. The kinematic data were collected while the patient produced 30 repetitions of the utterances "buy Bobby a poppy" and "sapapple." Each experimental trial required the patient to produce three consecutive repetitions of the utterance (i.e., "sapapple–sapapple–sapapple"). All the utterances were first produced using normal auditory feedback and then using the 80 msec delayed auditory feedback.

The kinematic data were digitized at 1 kHz per channel using a 500 Hz low-pass filter, a Data Translation A/D board (DT2801A), an IBM compatible computer, and CSpeech software. The data were transferred from CSpeech into the program ASYST (Asyst Software Technologies, Inc., 1989), which was used for the data processing and analysis procedures. Each of the lip and jaw movement channels were low-pass filtered at 30 Hz and differentiated in order to obtain velocity-time functions. The jaw signal was subtracted from the lower lip signal. The onset and termination points of the movements associated with the opening and closing gestures of the bilabial plosives were defined relative to the zero velocity crossings on the velocity–time functions. In the present study, only the closing gestures from the first "p" in sapapple are described. The following kinematic measures were obtained from the lip and jaw closing gestures: 1) movement duration, 2) maximum amplitude of movement, 3) peak velocity, 4) time to peak velocity (expressed as a percentage of the total movement time), 5) onset asynchrony (across structure differences in time of movement onset), and 6) peak velocity asynchrony (across structure differences in time of peak velocity).

RESULTS

Perceptual and Acoustic Data

Figure 1 indicates that, as the carrier sentence was repeated three times in succession, there was a tendency for the sentence to decrease in duration.

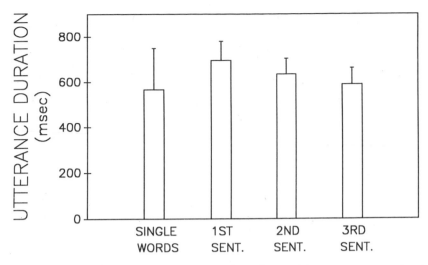

Figure 1. Average utterance durations for the single-word test and three-sentence test produced during the baseline (normal auditory feedback).

To compare these results with the patient's conversational speaking rate, the durations of the PIT sentences were converted to words per minute. Figure 2 indicates that the patient's rate of speech changed from a very rapid rate of approximately 350–400 words per minute, during base-

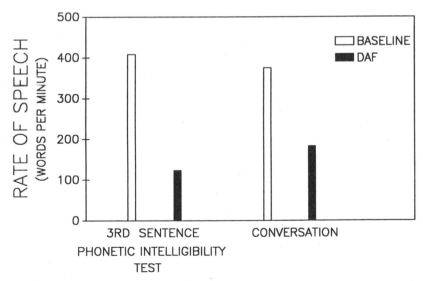

Figure 2. Average rate of speech (words per minute) obtained for the third test sentence and a 3-minute sample of conversational speech during the baseline and delayed auditory feedback.

line, to a significantly slower rate of speech that was roughly 150–200 words per minute during DAF.

Figure 3 indicates that the target word became significantly less intelligible across three consecutive repetitions of the carrier phrase. Thus, as speech rate increased over these repeated utterances, there was a corresponding decrease in intelligibility.

Figure 4 indicates that on both the PIT and the CAIDS the patient's intelligibility score increased from approximately 55% during baseline to approximately 95% during DAF.

The phonetic intelligibility test allowed the construction of a phonetic error profile based on eight phonetic categories (Figure 5). The most prominent phonetic errors were as follows:

1. Tense vowels were perceived as lax vowels.
2. Initial voiceless consonants were perceived as voiced consonants.
3. Affricates and fricatives were perceived as stops.
4. Stops were perceived as nasals.
5. Final consonants were perceived as nulls.
6. Consonant clusters were perceived as singletons.

Each error tended to become more frequent as the patient went from the first to the third production of the carrier sentence.

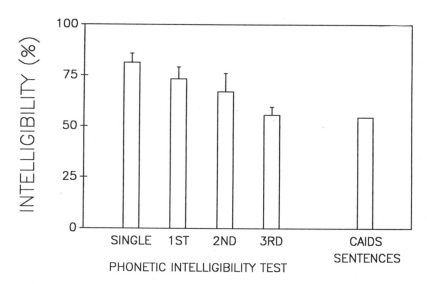

Figure 3. Average intelligibility scores (percentage of total words identified) for the single-word test, the three-sentence test, and the sentence portion of the CAIDS produced during baseline normal auditory feedback.

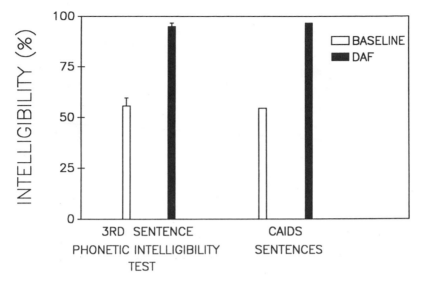

Figure 4. Average intelligibility scores (%) for the third test sentence and the sentence portion of the CAIDS produced during the baseline and delayed auditory feedback.

Figure 6 indicates that DAF was associated with a dramatic reduction in all of the patient's phonetic errors. Interestingly, the glottal/null error category continued to be present during DAF. This phonetic error may be a reflection of the patient's reduced voice quality, which did not seem to change with the use of delayed auditory feedback.

Examination of oscillograms and spectrograms provided additional information about the patient's intelligibility deficit and the effects of delayed auditory feedback (Figure 7). The baseline utterance was incorrectly perceived as "zip" rather than "sip," therefore, it was scored as a voicing error. Under DAF the word "sip" was correctly perceived. These waveforms suggest possible acoustic explanations for this voicing error. First, the amplitude and duration of frication noise in baseline was markedly reduced. Typically, voiced fricatives demonstrate a reduction in both frication duration and amplitude relative to voiceless fricatives. In addition, some voicing seems to have continued into the initial portion of the baseline fricative. This may have caused the listeners to perceive the fricative as voiced rather than voiceless.

Figure 8 is an example of the patient's production of the word "wax" during baseline and DAF. In the baseline, the word was perceived as "wack." This cluster/singleton error (ks/k) may have been related to the following acoustic features seen in the baseline condition: 1) a relatively short duration for the "ks" segment, 2) continuous voicing throughout the

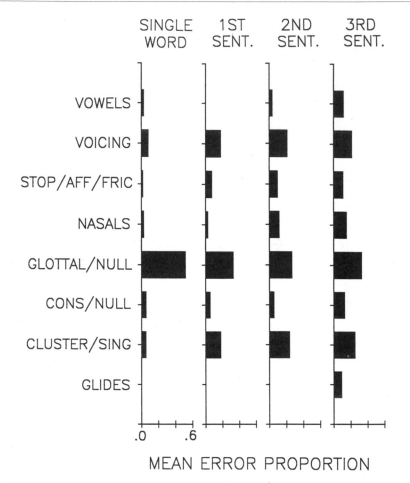

Figure 5. Phonetic error profiles for the single-word test and three-sentence test during the baseline normal auditory feedback.

"ks" segment, and 3) reduced intensity of frication noise and absence of a stop gap during the "ks" segment. In contrast, the patient's production of "ks" during DAF showed a clear stop gap and burst associated with the "k" segment and a relatively intense period of frication noise associated with the following "s" segment.

These spectrograms show that this patient's accelerated speech was characterized by a reduction in the distinctiveness of many acoustic features. This probably caused the listeners to misperceive and simplify the intended phonetic features. Under delayed auditory feedback, these phonetic features were more apparent and, as a result, were generally perceived correctly.

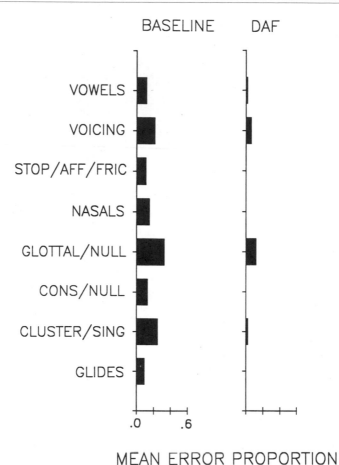

Figure 6. Phonetic error profiles for the three-sentence test produced during the baseline and delayed auditory feedback.

Kinematic Data

Figure 9 shows a tendency for the movements of the lower lip and jaw to become reduced gradually in amplitude over repeated productions of the utterance. In DAF, the lip and jaw movements were produced with greater amplitude and did not show a tendency to become reduced over repeated productions.

When baseline and DAF were compared statistically (Mann-Whitney Test $p < .05$) (Ryan, Joiner, & Ryan, 1985), it was found that the lower lip and jaw movements were produced with significantly larger average maximum displacements during DAF (Figure 10 a–d). In addition, the upper lip, lower lip, and jaw movements were all produced with signif-

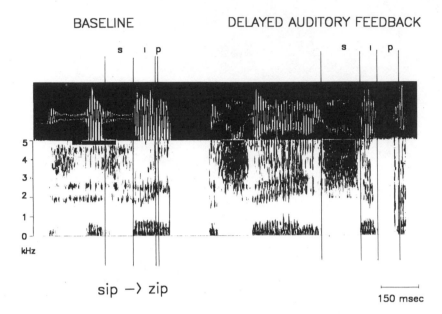

BASELINE DELAYED AUDITORY FEEDBACK

s   ı   p   s   ı   p

5
4
3
2
1
0
kHz

sip —⟩ zip

⊢————⊣
150 msec

Figure 7. Amplitude-time waveforms (upper panel) and 5 kz spectrograms (lower panel) for the patient's productions of the word "sip" in the three-sentence test. The "sip" sample on the left is from baseline normal auditory feedback, and the sample on the right is from the delayed auditory feedback. Both samples are on the same time scale.

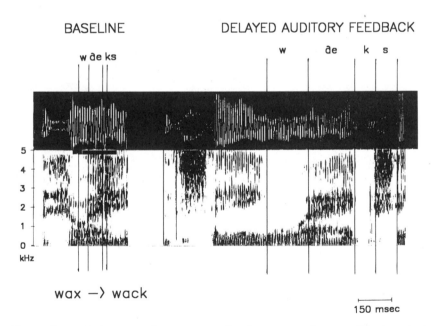

BASELINE DELAYED AUDITORY FEEDBACK

w ǝe ks   w   ǝe   k   s

5
4
3
2
1
0
kHz

wax —⟩ wack

⊢————⊣
150 msec

Figure 8. Amplitude-time waveforms (upper panel) and spectrograms (lower panel) for the patient's productions of the word "wax" in the three-sentence text. The "wax" sample on the left is from baseline normal auditory feedback, and the sample on the right is from the delayed auditory feedback.

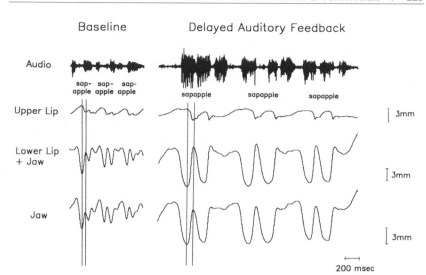

Figure 9. Examples of the lip and jaw movements for repeated productions of the utterance "sapapple" during baseline normal auditory feedback and delayed auditory feedback.

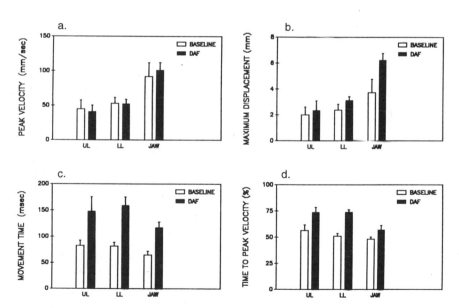

Figure 10. Average peak velocity values (a), average maximum displacement values (b), average movement time values (c), and average time to peak velocity (d) obtained from the upper lip, lower lip, and jaw movements during the baseline normal auditory feedback and delayed auditory feedback. All movements were obtained from the closing gestures produced during the first "p" in the utterance "sapapple."

icantly longer movement times and greater time to peak velocity values (%) during DAF. The average peak velocity for the lip and jaw movements were not significantly different across baseline and DAF.

In Figure 11, the upward bars indicate that the upper lip began moving before the lower lip, and downward bars indicate that the lower lip moved first. These onset asynchrony values indicate that during baseline, there was a very consistent order across structures for the timing of movement onsets. For every closing gesture, the onset of upper lip movement preceded the onset of lower lip movement, which preceded the onset of jaw movement. During DAF, this consistent pattern of movement onsets was disrupted. In DAF, more than half of the closing gestures were produced with the onset of lower lip movement preceding upper lip movement.

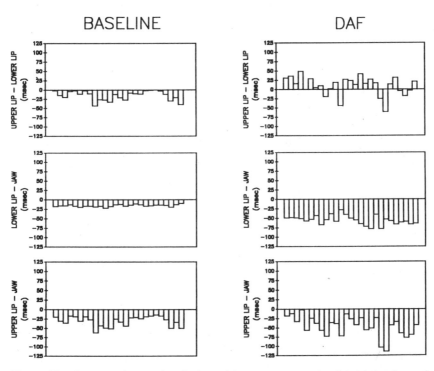

Figure 11. Onset asynchrony values for lip and jaw movements produced during baseline and delayed auditory feedback. All movements were obtained during the closing gesture of the first "p" in "sapapple." Values in the top panels represent the time of upper lip onset minus the time of lower lip onset. Middle panels represent lower lip onsets minus jaw onsets. The bottom panels represent the upper lip onsets minus the jaw onsets.

Figure 12 shows that there was a similar disruption in the timing between upper lip and lower lip peak velocities during DAF.

DISCUSSION

This study describes the effects of delayed auditory feedback on a number of perceptual/phonetic, acoustic, and kinematic correlates of accelerated speech. The perceptual and acoustic results indicate that, during normal auditory feedback, this patient showed a progressive increase in his rate of speech across consecutive repetitions of an utterance. This accelerating speech was found to have a very marked effect on intelligibility. With the introduction of delayed auditory feedback (80 msec), the patient's rate of speech was significantly reduced and there was corresponding improve-

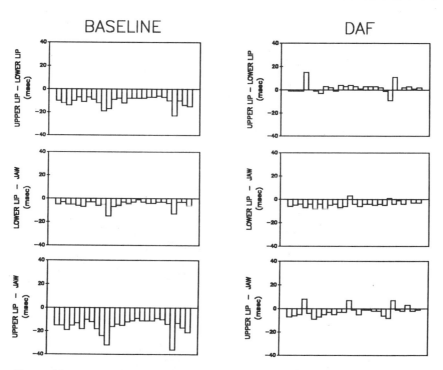

Figure 12. Peak velocity asynchrony values for lip and jaw movements produced during baseline and delayed auditory feedback. All movements were obtained during the closing gesture of the first "p" in "sapapple." Values in the top panels represent the time of upper lip peak velocity minus the time of lower lip peak velocity. Middle panels represent the time of lower lip peak velocity minus the time of jaw peak velocity. The bottom panels represent the time of upper lip peak velocity minus the time of jaw peak velocity.

ment in intelligibility. Specifically, under DAF, this patient reduced his rate of speech by approximately one half (from about 375 to fewer than 200 words per minute) and this was associated with a 40% increase in his intelligibility (from 55% to 95%). These results agree with previous studies that have reported slower and more intelligible speech in accelerating parkinsonian speakers treated with delayed auditory feedback (Downie et al., 1981; Hanson & Metter, 1981; Yorkston et al., 1988).

The results from the modified phonetic intelligibility test provided information about the phonetic distortions that contributed to the intelligibility deficit in this accelerated speaker. Many of the phonetic errors associated with the patient's accelerated speech seem to be related to a simplification of or reduction in the number of phonetic features transmitted. For example, consonant clusters were often heard as singletons, affricates were heard as stops, tense vowels were perceived as lax vowels, and final consonants often went undetected. In addition to these simplification errors, there were other phonetic errors related to incorrect perception of voicing and nasalization features. Results of the phonetic intelligibility test also indicated a marked reduction in the frequency of most phonetic errors during DAF. In particular, there were marked reductions in the frequency of vowel errors, voicing errors, stop/affricate/fricative errors, nasal errors, consonant/null errors, cluster/singleton errors, and glide errors.

Examination of the spectrograms indicated that this speaker's intelligibility deficit was not simply the result of an excessively rapid transmission of information. Instead, it seemed that many of the patient's phonetic errors were associated with a marked reduction in or absence of specific acoustic features. Under delayed auditory feedback, most of the expected phonetic and acoustic features were present and were produced fairly distinctly. As a result, the patient's speech intelligibility was markedly improved.

Previous kinematic studies have shown that the amplitude and peak velocity of lower lip and jaw movements are significantly reduced in individuals with dysarthria when compared to age-matched controls (Connor, Abbs, Cole, & Gracco, 1989; Forrest, Weismer, & Turner, 1989; Hirose, Kiritani, Ushijima, Yoshioka, & Sawashima, 1981). The finding that DAF produced an increase in movement amplitude while at the same time leaving peak velocity unchanged suggests that, in individuals with hypokinetic dysarthria and accelerated speech, certain movement parameters, such as the amplitude and duration of movement, may be more influenced by delayed auditory feedback than other parameters. In addition, it is possible that amplitude and duration play a greater role in the intelligibility deficit associated with accelerated speech than do other parameters, such as peak velocity.

Previous studies of nondisabled subjects have found consistent patterns in the timing of lip and jaw movement onsets and peak velocities (Gracco & Abbs, 1986). In particular, nondisabled subjects have been seen to begin the closing movements associated with bilabial stops by moving the upper lip first, then the lower lip, and the jaw last. In parkinsonian patients, this timing pattern has been reported to be disrupted. Moreover, this disruption has been suggested to be a reflection of the coordination deficit in hypokinetic dysarthria (Connor et al., 1989). Interestingly, the subject of this study was found to have lip and jaw coordination similar to that described for nondisabled subjects during the baseline condition. However, during DAF, the patient's coordination pattern changed to resemble the "dyscoordinated" pattern reported in other parkinsonian speakers. Such a finding brings into question the relative importance of this measure of coordination in Parkinson's and related disorders. It has been suggested by DeNil and Abbs (1991) and Tseng, McNeil, Adams, and Weismer (1990) that this pattern of oral coordination may be influenced significantly by the subject's rate of speech. Slower rates of speech, such as that produced by the patient using DAF in this study, seem to disrupt the normal stereotypic pattern of lip and jaw movements found for nondisabled subjects using faster rates of speech. Clearly, the information that can be gained from this measure of speech coordination in motor speech disorders needs to be re-evaluated.

Delayed auditory feedback has proved to be a practical, effective, and relatively long-term solution to the intelligibility deficit of the subject in this study. In fact, the patient has continued to use a portable, delayed auditory feedback device on a daily basis for almost 2 years and reports that its use is still essential for maintaining clarity in his conversational speech.

SUMMARY

The accelerated speech of one patient with an akinetic rigid syndrome suspected to be progressive supranuclear palsy was described using perceptual/phonetic, acoustic, and kinematic measures. The effect of treatment using a delayed auditory feedback of 80 msec was also described. Before DAF treatment, the patient's speech was very rapid (375 words/min), moderately intelligible (55%), and demonstrated a number of indistinct phonetic contrasts related to the production of tense/lax vowels, voiced/voiceless consonants, stop/fricative consonants, and cluster/singleton consonants. Under DAF treatment, the patient's speech became significantly slower (200 words/min), more intelligible (95%), and showed a reduction in the number of phonetic errors. Kinematic changes associated with DAF treatment included longer movement times, larger maximum displacements, and greater time to peak velocity values. The relative timing between lip and jaw movement onsets and peak velocities were also significantly affected by the patient's use of DAF.

REFERENCES

Asyst Software Technologies, Inc. (1989). *ASYST 3.1* [Computer program]. Rochester, New York.

Barlow, S., Cole, K., & Abbs, J. (1983). A new head-mounted lip–jaw movement transduction system for the study of motor speech disorders. *Journal of Speech and Hearing Research, 26,* 283–288.

Connor, N., Abbs, J., Cole, K., & Gracco, V. (1989). Parkinsonian deficits in serial multi-articulate movements for speech. *Brain, 112,* 997–1009.

Darley, F., Aronson, A., & Brown, J. (1975). *Motor speech disorders.* Philadelphia: W.B. Saunders.

DeNil, L., & Abbs, J. (1991). Influence of speaking rate on the upper lip, lower lip, and jaw peak, velocity sequencing during bilabial closing movements. *Acoustical Society of America. Journal. 89,* 845–849.

Downie, A., Low, J., & Lindsay, D. (1981). Speech disorder in Parkinsonism: Usefulness of delayed auditory feedback in selected cases. *British Journal of Disorders of Communication, 16,* 135–139.

Forrest, K., Weismer, G., & Turner, G. (1989). Kinematic, acoustic, and perceptual analyses of connected speech produced by Parkinsonian and normal geriatric adults. *Journal of the Acoustical Society of America, 85,* 2608–2622.

Gracco, V., & Abbs, J. (1986). Variant and invariant characteristics of speech movements. *Experimental Brain Research, 65,* 156–166.

Hanson, W., & Metter, E. (1981). DAF as instrumental treatment for dysarthria in progressive supranuclear palsy: A case report. *Journal of Speech and Hearing Disorders, 45,* 268–276.

Hanson, W., & Metter, E. (1983). DAF speech rate modification in Parkinson's disease: A report of two cases. In W. R. Berry (Ed.), *Clinical dysarthria* (pp. 231–251). San Diego: College–Hill.

Hirose, H., Kiritani, S., Ushijima, T., Yoshioka, H., & Sawashima, M. (1981). Patterns of dysarthric movements in patients with Parkinsonism. *Folia Phoniatrica, 33,* 204–215.

Kent, R., Weismer, G., Kent, J., & Rosenbek, J. (1989). Toward explanatory intelligibility testing in dysarthria. *Journal of Speech and Hearing Disorders, 54,* 482–499.

Milenkovic, P. (1990). *CSpeech.* [Computer program]. Department of Electrical and Computer Engineering, University of Wisconsin-Madison.

Ryan, B.F., Joiner, B.L., & Ryan, T.A. (18985). *Minitab handbook.* Boston: Duxbury Press.

Tseng, C., McNeil, M.R., Adams, S.G., & Weismer, G. (1990). *Effects of speaking rate on bilabial (a)synchrony in neurogenic populations.* Paper presented at the American Speech-Language-Hearing Association Conference, Seattle, WA.

Yorkston, K., Beukelman, D., & Bell, K. (1988). *Clinical management of dysarthric speakers.* Boston: College-Hill.

Yorkston, K., Beukelman, D., & Traynor, C. (1984). *Computerized assessment of intelligibility of dysarthric speech.* Austin, TX: PRO-ED.

Chapter 17

Effects of Syllable Characteristics and Training on Speaking Rate in a Child with Dysarthria Secondary to Near-Drowning

Megan M. Hodge and Susan D. Hall

THE IMPETUS FOR this investigation was a request to develop a treatment plan for an 11-year-old boy with dysarthria secondary to brain damage incurred in a near-drowning accident 6 years previously. The major factor interfering with his communicative interactions in classroom and social activities was his extremely slow speaking rate (less than one syllable per second) which resulted in long durations of his conversational turns. Previous interventions to compensate for or increase his slow rate had limited success, which was partly attributed to limited self-monitoring abilities. From a speech motor control perspective, the important question was, "Does this child have the physiologic resources to increase his speaking rate?" A literature search revealed no information describing speech outcomes with this subject population. Furthermore, methods for modifying speaking rate in adults only were found. This chapter docu-

This project was supported by funds from the Office of Research Services, Glenrose Rehabilitation Hospital, Edmonton, Alberta, Canada. We express appreciation to Susan Crack, Heather Hancock, and Peter Schoenberg for their assistance.

ments the procedures used to determine this child's potential to increase his speaking rate.

Speaking rate (typically measured in words or syllables per unit time) is the speed at which speech sound sequences are produced. Rate expressed in syllables per second (sps) implies measurement within a phrase without pauses and periodic inspirations, whereas rate expressed in syllables per minute (spm) includes both pauses and periodic inspirations. For children 10–11 years old, mean spontaneous speaking rates of 4.93 sps were reported by Haselager, Slis, and Rietveld (1991) and mean oral reading rates of 3.52 sps were reported by Hoit, Hixon, Watson, and Morgan (1990). Speaking rates vary for an individual speaker depending on speaking context, speaker state, phonetic content, and utterance length. Haselager et al. (1991) reported that for groups of children without speech disabilities, 5–11 years, speaking rates for simple consonant-vowel (CV) syllables (e.g., "ba," "da") were greater than for more complex syllable shapes such as CVC (e.g., "hat") or CCVC (e.g., "stop"). Generally for these subjects, as the number of syllables in an utterance increased, speaking rate also increased. Several temporal components of speech production contribute to speaking rate (Yorkston, Beukelman, & Bell, 1988). One is the speed of articulatory movements as muscles alter the size and shape of the vocal tract, producing the sequences of consonant and vowel sounds that make up the speech signal. Second is the duration of steady-state portions of utterances where no movement is occurring (sounds such as the midportion of monophthongal vowels, continuant consonant sounds such as /s/, or when the vocal tract is closed to build up air pressure for a stop consonant such as /t/). When measured in spm, the third component of speaking rate is number and duration of pauses that mark syntactical boundaries and that typically co-occur with inspirations. For a speaker with dysarthria, rates for more complex syllable content may be substantially reduced, compared to speech with simple syllable content, because of the additional time and effort required to produce a greater number of articulatory gestures in more complex syllables (R. Kent, personal communication, May 8, 1991). Therefore, one objective of this investigation was to describe the effects of different syllable characteristics on the subject's speaking rate.

When speaking rates are slowed substantially, disturbances in stress patterning, intonation, and rate-rhythm typically result. These prosodic disturbances reduce the naturalness or "acceptability" of speech and may increase the degree of handicap experienced by a speaker with dysarthria (Yorkston et al., 1988). Moreover, the quality of social–verbal interactions can be affected adversely by the longer time the listener needs to receive the speaker's message and by disturbances in the rhythm and synchrony of speaker turn-taking (Blackstone, 1990). Adverse listener behaviors include avoiding the speaker as a conversational partner, interrupting or completing the speaker's utterance, or aborting the conversational interaction. Thus, an important goal to improve both the quality and quantity of spoken interactions in speakers with dysarthria who are intelligible, but who have substantially reduced speaking rates, is to decrease the duration of their spoken messages. This may be accomplished by: 1) decreasing pause time and syllable duration in order to increase speaking rate, and 2) improving production-monitoring skills to minimize the number of words required for successful message transmission in various contexts. This investigation focused on training to increase speaking rate by eliminating intrusive within-utterance inspiratory pauses and decreasing syllable durations.

Yorkston and Beukelman (1981) described rate control procedures for four adult speakers with dysarthria. Treatment sequences were based on procedures to enhance speech intelligibility and prosody by initially slowing speaking rate to maximize intelligibility. As speakers improved, a compromise was made between intelligibility and rate—maintaining a target level of speech intelligibility, while maximizing speaking rate. Two rate-control techniques described by Yorkston and Beukelman (1981) were *rhythmic cuing* and *oscilloscopic feedback*. In rhythmic cuing, a clinician indicates the pace at which words should be spoken by pointing to them as they are said. Stressed syllables are cued more slowly than unstressed syllables. Speakers are instructed to follow the rhythm. In the oscilloscopic feedback procedure, a microphone is used to record the acoustic waveform of the speaker's utterance, which is displayed as a time-by-amplitude tracing on the face of an oscilloscope. If a storage oscilloscope is used, the clinician can record a model of the utterance at target rate. The speaker than attempts to match this target rate. The time-base of the display can be altered so that the speaker must learn to fit the utterance into shorter or longer time periods by increasing or decreasing speaking rate. Berry and Goshorn (1983) described the effective use of immediate visual feedback by an oscilloscope to decrease speaking rate and increase intelligibility in an adult with ataxic dysarthria. These authors observed that:

> Speech therapy with dysarthric adults generally relies upon the clinician's judgment of patient responses. A more favorable treatment plan would allow the patient to monitor and change speech behaviors as efficiently as possible. A biofeedback program in which a patient receives instantaneous and continuous information about his [or her] neuromotor behavior may be the most desirable for shaping behavior toward a desired goal. (p. 253)

The treatment procedures used in the present investigation combined "modeling," using a modification of the rhythmic cuing technique, with real-time visual feedback of amplitude and durational aspects in the speech acoustic waveform provided by the SpeechViewer system (International Business Machines, 1989). The SpeechViewer system is a combination of hardware and software designed for speech training. It uses a computer to record a speech signal digitally and convert into interactive graphic displays of the duration, amplitude, and frequency features of the recorded utterance. It uses dynamic visual effects to motivate clients and to provide feedback of key features of speech models. The Pitch and Loudness Patterning module in SpeechViewer provides a real-time, time-by-amplitude display similar to that provided by a storage oscilloscope. A choice of three time-bases (4, 8, and 12 seconds) is available. The split-screen mode permits a target utterance to be displayed for the client to use as a model. Digital audio playback of the recorded signal can be synchronized with the visual display, which enables the client to compare his or her production with the clinician's model of the target utterance. Thus, SpeechViewer provides immediate, visual displays of utterance durations in a time-controlled mode, and simultaneous auditory and visual playback of recorded utterances. It was thought that this system would motivate the subject to "beat the computer clock" and provide him with immediate, specific information about his success in meeting rate training targets.

In summary, the purpose of this investigation was to determine if an 11-year-old boy with dysarthria characterized by an extremely slow speaking rate could increase his rate when given specific training to decrease the frequency of intrusive within-utterance inspirations and to shorten syllable durations. Treatment procedures incorporated computer software that provided immediate and interpretable visual displays of these speech features in a time-controlled mode. It was hypothesized that if the subject had the physiological potential to increase speaking rate, this potential would be maximized by an approach that was motivating and that provided immediate, specific feedback and knowledge of results (Schmidt, 1988). If the subject was unable to increase speaking rate, then other strategies to improve his communication efficiency should be developed and evaluated.

In addition to the effects of the training procedures, the effects of two syllable characteristics on the subject's speaking rate were also investigated. These were syllable shape (open and closed) and number of syllables in a word (mono- and multisyllabic). It was predicted that for utterances of the same syllable length: 1) utterances containing open syllables only would be produced at faster rates than those containing a combination of open and closed syllables because of the additional time required to produce the greater number of articulatory gestures in closed syllables, and 2) utterances containing a combination of mono- and multisyllabic words would be produced at faster rates than those containing monosyllabic words only.

METHOD

Subject

The subject was an 11-year-old boy who suffered hypoxic encephalopathy as a result of a warm water near-drowning accident at the age of 5 years. A CT scan performed 4 weeks postaccident revealed progressive ventricular dilation and enlargement of the cortical sulci. An MRI evaluation performed on the subject at 6½ years postaccident revealed a mild enlargement of the lateral ventricles; however, no focal lesions were evident in the cortex, cerebellum, or brainstem. At the time of this investigation, the subject was ambulatory with residual mild ataxia and spasticity in the limbs. He had language-processing and memory difficulties with an overall language age equivalent of 8 years on the Clinical Evaluation of Language Fundamentals—Revised (Semel, Wiig, & Secord, 1987), and auditory–visual attention problems that hindered his development of functional reading and writing skills. He was enrolled in a school for children with learning disabilities.

These findings and the subject's general level of function are similar to those described for a subgroup of children by Asano, Ieshima, Kisa, and Ohatani (1991) who investigated early serial CT findings and later outcomes in children following near-drowning. In this subgroup, CT images did not show atrophy of the pons after 2 months, although enlargement of the cerebral sulci and the lateral and third ventricles was observed at 3–4 weeks following hospital admission. The authors stated:

> The prognosis for all of these patients was that they would be able to walk and speak after two to three years. Although their walking was ataxic and they lacked the ability to make elaborate movements with their arms, these patients did not suffer from any obvious pyramidal or cerebellar symptoms. Dystonia was recognized in one of these cases but no other cases of involuntary movement disorders were seen. The extent of mental retardation was minor. . . . (English translation, p. 230)

Specific information about speech motor outcomes was not provided by Asano et al. (1991).

Pre-Experimental Function Prior to this investigation, the subject's mean speaking rate in a sentence imitation task was 0.85 sps. On this task, he produced an average of 2.5 syllables per breath (range of one to four syllables per breath), compared to a mean of nine syllables per breath expected for nondisabled boys of his age (Hoit et al., 1990). His prosody in conversational speech had a "dissociated pattern" (Kent & Rosenbek, 1982), characterized by a regularity in syllable durations and a resetting of fundamental frequency after every one or two words. His prosody was described by some listeners as a sing-song pattern. His best maximum phonation time for a sustained vowel was 16 seconds, within normal limits for his age. He had difficulty grading the loudness of his speech and, when asked to speak loudly, his voice quality became harsh and rough. His speech intelligibility for a 100-word conversational speech sample, judged by a familiar listener using a word identification task, was 95%. His mean speech intelligibility score on a single-word test (Kent, Weismer, Kent, & Rosenbek, 1989), when three nonfamiliar listeners transcribed audio recordings of his single words, was 50%. Error contrasts on this single-word test included high/low and tense/lax vowels, consonant voicing, affricate/fricative, singleton/cluster, initial glottal/null, and liquid/glide. Redundancy of his lengthy utterances in conversational speech seemed to increase his intelligibility for familiar listeners substantially.

In summary, the subject had three notably abnormal speech behaviors.

1. His mean speaking rate was extremely slow, less than one quarter of the expected norm.
2. He had an unusual style of breathing when talking, characterized by very short breath groups and inspirations at inappropriate places, such as within vowels, words, and phrases.
3. He had unusual stress patterning, intonation, and rate-rhythm, characterized by stereotypic syllable durations and pitch patterns, and poor control over vocal effort and quality. Spastic-ataxic dysarthria was diagnosed based on these speech characteristics and the physical signs in his limbs. However, as noted, no focal lesions in the cortex, corticobulbar pathways, or cerebellum were evident on MRI scans.

Prognostic Considerations Three observations seemed positive in regard to the prognosis for speech improvement.

1. He responded to stimuli to induce more natural sounding prosody on short imitation tasks.
2. Despite his use of very short breath groups, his maximum phonation time was within normal limits. This suggested that he had adequate breath support to produce a greater number of syllables per breath.
3. He seemed very interested in using SpeechViewer to obtain feedback about his speech.

However, several factors seemed negative in regard to his potential for speech improvement.

1. Length of time post-onset of the speech disorder. The patient described by Yorkston and Beukelman (1981), who was able to increase speaking rate after an initial period of rate reduction was in the post-onset period when spontaneous recovery was expected (less than a

year). Similar results might not be expected for a patient whose recovery had stabilized, such as the subject described here, who was 6 years post-onset.

2. The effects of accompanying residual sequelae of the subject's brain damage (including attention and memory deficits and increased response latency) on his ability to process instructions, perform speaking tasks under time pressure, and interpret visual feedback.

3. The tendency for spasticity and ataxia to be resistive to behavioral training (K. Yorkston, personal communication, September 2, 1992).

Procedures

All sessions took place in a sound-treated booth. Audio recordings of all test utterances in each session were made using a Sony electret condensor microphone (Model 144) clipped to the subject's shirtfront and connected to a Sony TCRX-410 stereo cassette recording deck located outside the sound booth.

Syllable Characteristics   Three types of utterances were used. Type I contained only open (V, CV, VC) syllables and had both mono- and multisyllabic words (e.g., "Buy a puppy"; "A lazy goalie"; "See the tiny baby"; "Say hello to my new buddy."). Type II contained open and closed syllables and had both mono- and multisyllabic words (e.g., "Pick the turtle"; "Open the blue box"; "More peanut butter, please"; "My summer camp is in August."). Type III contained open and closed syllables and had only monosyllabic words (e.g., "He said stop now"; "Do you like to skip?"; "Plant the seeds in the pot"; "Is the lake warm or cold this year?"). Master pools of 40 utterances were developed for each of the three utterance types for four utterance lengths (four, five, six, and eight syllables) for a total of 12 master pools. Test utterances were selected randomly from these master pools for each training session. This was done to increase the interest level of the speech-training material and to control for utterance-specific practice effects. A comparison of Type I versus Type II utterances permitted comparison of speaking rates for open versus a combination of open and closed syllable shapes. A comparison of Type III versus Type II utterances permitted comparison of speaking rates for monosyllabic versus a combination of mono- and multisyllabic words.

Dependent Variables   Two dependent variables were measured in each session. The first was the percentage of utterance trials that contained no within-utterance inspirations. The occurrence and location of within-utterance inspirations were identified on a transcript of the test utterances by an observer as the subject produced each utterance. These locations were rechecked later by a second observer using the tape-recorded utterances. The second dependent variable was the percentage of utterance trials that met the speaking rate criterion in sps. The speaking rate for each utterance trial produced per session was measured from the audio recordings. *CSpeech* (Milenkovic, 1990), a speech waveform analysis software package, was used with a microcomputer and associated signal-processing equipment to obtain utterance duration in milliseconds. This duration was then divided by the number of syllables in the utterance to provide speaking rate in sps. Remeasurement of 10% of the utterances indicated that the mean measurement error was less than 0.01 sps, so rate measures were rounded to the nearest 0.01 sps.

Design

A time-series, changing criterion design (Ottenbacher & York, 1984) was used. Data were collected for 4 baseline sessions and 12 training sessions over a four-week period. The changing criterion was the number of sylla-bles in the utterance tokens. This ranged from four to eight syllables. For inspiratory loci, the objective was to produce utterances of increasing syllable number without within-utterance inspirations. For speaking rate, the objective was to produce utterances of increasing syllable number within a constant time period. The period selected was the 4-second screen length in the SpeechViewer Pitch and Loudness Patterning module. This provided a real-time, time-by-amplitude display of the speech signal with a 4-second screen sweep. To fit within this time period, four-syllable utterances must be produced at a minimum rate of 1.0 sps, five-syllable utterances must be produced at a minimum rate of 1.25 sps, six-syllable utterances must be produced at a minimum rate of 1.50 sps, and so on.

Data were plotted separately for each utterance type. For each of the two dependent variables, generally when a percentage of 80% or greater of utterance trials met the criterion for at least three consecutive sessions, the criterion was changed to the next syllable length. However, this rule was not followed in all instances. The first criterion utterance length selected for training was four syllables for both dependent variables.

Baseline Prior to treatment, the subject attended four sessions so that baseline measures of speaking rate and the two dependent variables could be obtained for the three utterance types, in two conditions, *no instruction* and *fast instruction*. In the no instruction condition, he was asked to repeat the test utterances after the examiner. In the fast instruction condition, he was asked to repeat each utterance as fast as he could. The no instruction condition always preceded the fast instruction condition. In both conditions, the utterances were presented by the investigator, using a natural prosodic pattern at target rates between three-and-one-half and four sps, cued by the flashing light on a digital metronome. In each baseline session, for each instruction condition, two utterances were randomly selected from the master pools of four-, six-, and eight-syllable utterances for each of the three utterance types (2 instruction conditions × 2 utterances × 3 syllable lengths × 3 utterance types for a total of 36 utterance tokens).

Training Two different treatments were administered in each of the 12 training sessions. The utterance tokens used in each intervention session were selected randomly from the appropriate master pools of utterance types and syllable lengths.

Treatment A: Elimination of Within-Utterance Inspirations (No Time Pressure) At the beginning of each session, the subject was reminded that he should take a breath just before speaking each test utterance, and that he should try to complete the utterance without taking another breath. This was followed by a warm-up period of about 10 minutes during which the subject practiced inspiring just prior to making utterances of various syllable lengths (sequences of numbers or letters of the alphabet) in turn-taking activities with one of the investigators. After each practice utterance, the subject was given feedback about whether he had remembered to take a breath just before speaking and whether he had inspired part way through the utterance. Praise was given for each practice utterance that had a pre-utterance inspiration and no within-utterance inspirations. After this warm-up period, the training/test utterances were introduced. Five utterances of each type were presented. Immediately following presentation of each utterance token, the investigator said, "breathe," placing her hand on the child's chest to cue an inspiration. The child's production of the utterance was recorded using the SpeechViewer Pitch and Loudness Patterning module and then was played back so that the presence of any within-utterance (intrusive) inspirations could be identified. The subject was praised when he produced an utterance without intrusive inspirations. For criterion syllable number, the number of successful trials for each utterance type was graphed on a chart for each phase. Prior to each set of utterance trials, the subject was shown the graph of his previous performance and encouraged to surpass it.

Treatment B: Rate Training To Increase the Number of Syllables Produced in Four Seconds This treatment always followed Treatment A in the sessions. During a 15-minute warm up period, the subject was given opportunities to practice: 1) grading and controlling the loudness of repeated syllables using the Loudness Awareness and Pitch and Loudness Patterning module in SpeechViewer, and 2) decreasing syllable durations in one- and two-syllable words by using visual feedback of syllable duration provided by the split-screen display in the Pitch and Loudness patterning module together with a hand signal to cue "finish the syllable now." Following the warm-up period, treatment procedures specific to meeting the rate criterion were initiated. These procedures were based on a modification of rhythmic cuing (provided by an auditory model of an utterance token presented by the trainer) and oscilloscopic feedback (provided by the 4-second display in the Pitch and Loudness Patterning module in SpeechViewer) techniques. The investigator presented each utterance token at a target rate between 3.5 to 4.0 sps with natural prosody, so that syllable stress patterns were preserved. Immediately following presentation of the utterance, the investigator instructed the subject to "Wait," "Think," "Breathe." These cue words were selected to reduce the subject's response impulsivity, to increase his focus on controlling production, and to remind him to inspire just before speaking. Each of the subject's productions was recorded and displayed in real time on the time-by-amplitude display in the Pitch and Loudness Patterning module. After recording, each production was played back so that the subject could listen and see if he has been successful in fitting his utterance into the 4-second screen. The subject was praised when he completed his utterance within the 4-second limit. If he exceeded the time limit, he was asked how he could change his production to fit it within the time limit. His responses were discussed in relation to the training objectives of eliminating intrusive inspirations, controlling loudness, and shortening syllable durations. As in Treatment A, the number of his successful trials for each utterance type was graphed on a chart for each syllable number criterion. Prior to each set of utterance trials, he was shown the graph of his previous performance and encouraged to surpass it.

RESULTS AND DISCUSSION

Effects of Instruction Condition, Utterance Type, and Syllable Length on Speaking Rate

The means and standard deviations shown in Figure 1 seem similar across instruction condition and session, suggesting that rate measures in baseline were relatively stable with negligible differences between instruction conditions. Across the no instruction condition in the baseline sessions, the subject demonstrated a slight increase in speaking rate (0.98 sps–1.09 sps), suggesting that practice repeating the sentences alone, with no feedback, had some effect on increasing his rate. It is also of interest that in the final baseline session, his rate in the no instruction condition surpassed his rate in the fast condition. In the fast instruction condition, it was observed that the subject greatly increased his effort level with resulting loss of control over loudness and voice quality. For the no instruction condition, this loss of control was not as evident, even when utterances in this condition were produced at higher rates than those in the fast condition. Thus, it seemed that he could increase his rate slightly beyond his typical values without losing control of his laryngeal/respiratory mechanism. The addi-

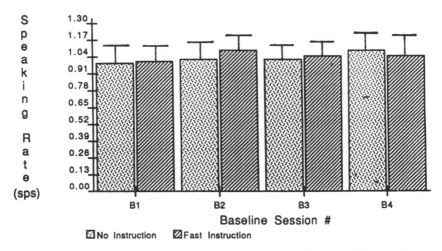

Figure 1. Comparison of speaking rates averaged across utterance type and syllable length for the no instruction (NI) and fast instruction (FI) conditions in the four baseline (B) sessions.

tional effort that the subject made in response to the word, fast, may have served to decrease his rate compared to the rate increase he experienced from cumulative practice in repeating test utterances.

Mean speaking rates (sps) for the four-syllable utterances of each type are shown in Figure 2 for four different conditions. These conditions were used for comparison because for each utterance type, utterances of four

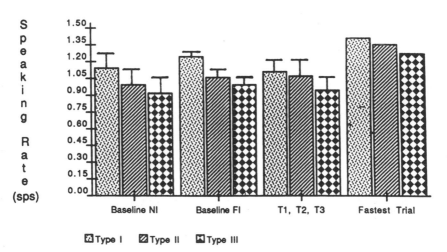

Figure 2. Comparison of mean speaking rates for the 4-syllable Type I, II, and III utterances in four conditions: 1) baseline—no instruction (Baseline NI); 2) baseline—fast instruction (Baseline FI); 3) first three treatment sessions (T1, T2, T3); and 4) the fastest utterance trial across the four baseline and first three treatment sessions (Fastest Trial).

syllables were produced in these seven sessions (four baseline and first three treatment sessions). In all conditions, mean rates for Type I utterances (open syllables, mono- and multisyllabic words) were higher than those for Type II utterances (open and closed syllables, mono- and multisyllabic words), and rates for Type II utterances were higher than those for Type III utterances (open and closed syllables, monosyllabic words). This same pattern was also observed for the six- and eight-syllable utterances in the baseline sessions. Mean speaking rates for the four-, six- and eight-syllable utterances in the baseline sessions, averaged across utterance type and instruction condition were very similar, 1.05 sps (SD = 0.16), 1.03 sps (SD = 0.14) and 1.01 sps (SD = 0.10) respectively for the four-, six- and eight-syllable lengths. Thus, although utterance type seemed to influence the subject's speaking rate, utterance length seemed to have a negligible effect. As predicted: 1) utterances containing open syllables only were produced at faster rates than utterances containing a combination of open and closed syllables, and 2) utterances containing monosyllabic words only were produced at slower rates than utterances containing a combination of mono- and multisyllabic words. Unlike the children with no speech disabilities described by Haselager et al. (1991), this subject did not produce utterances of greater syllable number at faster speaking rates.

Effects of Training To Eliminate Within-Utterance Breaths

Figure 3 shows that for the open syllable only (Type I) utterances, there was an initial decrement in performance when the criterion utterance length was increased from four to five syllables, followed by an improvement in performance over time. The next decrement in performance did not occur until the introduction of eight-syllable utterances. For the other utterance types, it took longer to establish consistent performance at the four-syllable criterion, but once established, performance did not fall off until the eight-syllable criterion was introduced. These results support the observation that the subject was able to reduce the occurrence of within-utterance inspirations in the treatment sessions, on utterances of successively greater syllable number.

Figure 4 shows that for all utterance types, performance in the last treatment session was improved, compared to baseline performance.

Effect of Training To Increase the Number of Syllables Produced in Four Seconds

It can be seen in Figure 5 that the subject met the criterion to move from utterances of four syllables (1.00 sps) to five syllables (1.25 sps) for Type I and II utterances, but not Type III. Performance was best for Type I utterances, with the criterion length of five syllables introduced after just

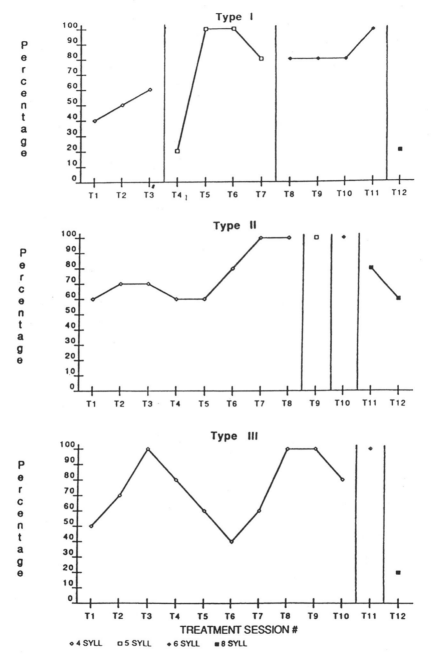

Figure 3. Percentage of utterances in the breath-training condition in each treatment session that met the criterion of no within-utterance inspiration.

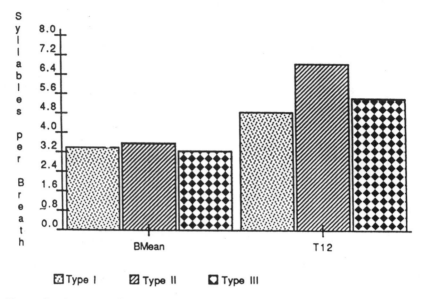

Figure 4. Comparison of the mean number of syllables per breath for the eight-syllable utterances of each type in the baseline (B) sessions and the final treatment session (T12).

three treatment sessions. The next best performance was for Type II utterances, with the criterion length of five syllables introduced after eight treatment sessions. Although performance for the Type III utterances did not improve to the level required to introduce the five-syllable criterion, an improvement in performance within the four-syllable criterion phase was apparent.

The solid symbols in Figure 5 show the percentage of utterances produced in the time-pressure rate-training condition that contained no within-utterance breaths. The positive trend of these solid lines in each phase for each utterance type suggests that the subject transferred the breath-training treatment to the rate-training treatment. In Figure 5, the tendency for the data points for rate and breath criterion to follow a similar pattern suggests that elimination of inspirations contributed to increased speaking rate.

Figure 6 shows that for all three types rates were higher for utterance tokens that did not contain inspirations. To determine if elimination of within-utterance breaths accounted solely for the subject's improved performance in meeting the rate criterion in treatment, the mean speaking rates for all utterance types that did not contain a within-utterance breath in each training session were plotted in Figure 7. Using a celeration line technique (Ottenbacher, 1986), a slight positive slope is evident, suggest-

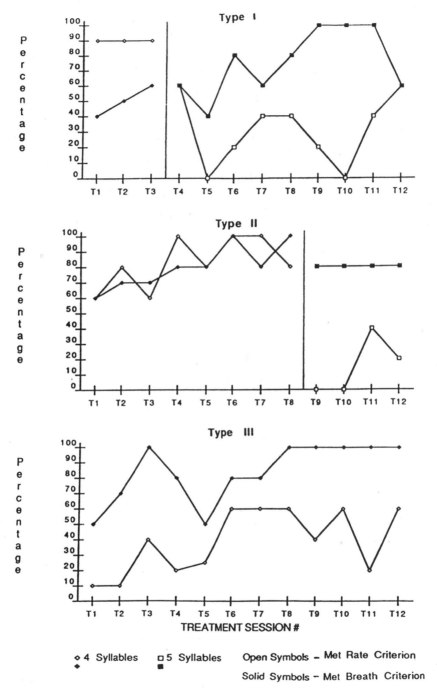

Figure 5. Percentages of utterances of each type in the time pressure rating-training condition that: 1) met the rate criterion for the phase; that is, produced within four seconds (open symbols); and 2) contained no within-utterance breaths (solid symbols) in each treatment session.

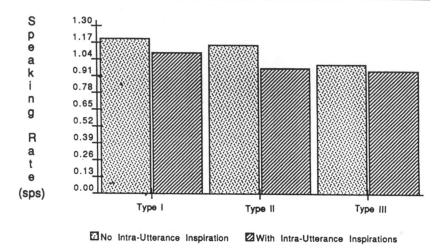

Figure 6. Comparison of mean speaking rates in the rate-training (time-pressure) condition for the three utterance types that did and did not contain within-utterance inspirations. Rates have been pooled across the 12 training sessions.

ing that decreases in syllable duration also contributed, although in a small way, to increased rates.

Table 1 provides a comparison of the subject's speaking rates at several points in the investigation. Mean speaking rate for all syllable tokens of each utterance type are for the first and the fourth baseline sessions (pooled across syllable length and instruction condition) and for the time-pressure condition in the final (12th) treatment session. These data include both utterances that contained within-utterance inspirations and

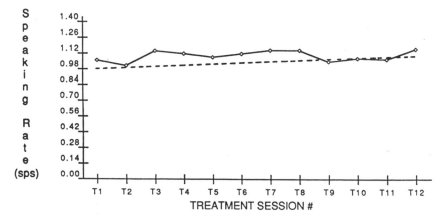

Figure 7. Mean speaking rates for all utterance types that did not contain a within-utterance breath in the time-pressure training condition. A celeration line (dashed line) has been fit to the data points.

Table 1. Comparison of mean speaking rates in baseline with the final treatment session

	Utterance type			
	Type I (sps)	Type II (sps)	Type III (sps)	M (sps)
First baseline session	1.10	0.91	0.95	0.99
SD	0.10	0.10	0.13	0.14
Fourth baseline session	1.19	1.07	0.94	1.07
SD	0.17	0.09	0.07	0.16
Last treatment session	1.22	1.16	1.07	1.15
SD	0.11	0.13	0.19	0.16

Speaking rates in the baseline sessions are averaged across instruction condition and syllable number.

those that did not. First, for all three utterance types, mean speaking rate was higher at the end of treatment than in the final baseline session. However, the proportion of total rate increase observed in the baseline and treatment phases varied with utterance type. Type I utterances demonstrated an increase of 0.12 sps between the first baseline and final treatment session. However, 75% (0.09 sps) of this increase is between the first and fourth baseline sessions, suggesting that treatment had a minimal effect on increasing rate for Type I utterances beyond the practice afforded in baseline. Type II utterances demonstrated an increase of 0.25 sps between the first baseline and final treatment session. Again, a greater proportion of this change (64% or 0.16 sps) occurred between the first and fourth baseline sessions than between the final baseline and final treatment session. Type III utterances demonstrated a change of 0.12 sps between the first baseline and the final treatment session. Type III differed from the other two utterance types in that 100% of the rate increase occurred between the final baseline and final treatment session. This pattern of results suggests that the training procedures had the least effect on Type I utterances and the greatest effect on Type III utterances.

The fastest utterance trial produced for each utterance type during the investigation is shown in Table 2. None of these utterance trials contained a within-utterance inspiration. Speaking rates for these trials ranged from 1.40 to 1.73 sps for a mean of 1.52 sps. This mean maximal speaking rate, which is thought to represent the upper limit of the sub-

Table 2. Fastest utterance trials produced by the subject in the investigation

	Utterance	Length (syllables)	Rate (sps)
Type I	A boy ate toffee.	5	1.73
Type II	At the bottom.	4	1.40
Type III	He is the best.	4	1.42
M			1.52

ject's physiological capacity, is 0.53 sps greater than his first baseline session mean of 0.99 sps, which represents about a 52% increase in rate. This mean maximal rate is about 43% (1.52 compared to 3.52 sps) of that expected for his age.

CONCLUSIONS

Syllable Characteristics

The results for syllable shape (open only versus open and closed) and number of syllables in a word (monosyllabic only versus mono- and multi-syllabic) suggest that for utterances of equal syllable number, closed syllables and monosyllabic words act to decrease rate. As with the children with no speech disabilities described by Haselager et al. (1991), the subject had faster speaking rates for utterances with open syllables only versus those with a combination of open and closed syllables. The subject also demonstrated faster rates for utterances containing mono- and multisyllabic words versus those containing monosyllabic words only. One interpretation of this finding is that despite his prolongation of syllables within a word, he could alter duration for relative syllable stress. Inspection of several of his multisyllabic utterances supported this interpretation. When the multisyllabic word did not occur in utterance final position, the syllable that would typically receive primary stress was longer in duration than the other syllables. Generalization of this strategy to his spontaneous speech should improve the naturalness of his prosody. An unexpected finding was that the subject did not produce utterances of greater syllable number at faster speaking rates. One possibility is that utterances of increasing syllable number placed an additional load on his speech production system that limited speaking rate. These results indicate that syllable characteristics should be considered and controlled in stimuli used to measure speaking rate.

Training Procedures

Observations Regarding Use of the SpeechViewer The auditory–visual processing deficits that were reported to interfere with the subject's ability to learn to read did not seem to interfere with his ability to learn to interpret the time-by-amplitude display in the Pitch and Loudness Patterning module in SpeechViewer. Throughout the training sessions, the subject indicated, via both solicited and unsolicited comments, that he was interpreting the visual feedback on the SpeechViewer screen in several beneficial ways. He could control his speech to produce the same syllable at different durations, primarily by reducing the duration of medial and final continuant sounds. He reliably indicated whether a syllable was relatively longer or shorter than another on the screen display and whether he fit an utterance trial within the 4-second screen. Using the screen display, he could indicate if one syllable was of greater amplitude than another and could grade his effort to produce the same syllable at various loudness levels. In later sessions, when he observed that his voice was too loud or rough, as shown by the on-line relative amplitude pattern displayed on the screen, he modified vocal effort and quality to a more appropriate level. However, as expected from his history, the subject had a short attention span, memory constraints, and variable effort level from session to session, which may have contributed to the performance variability observed in the dependent measures across treatment sessions. A problem was encountered with the Pitch and Loudness Patterning module in SpeechViewer; in order to activate the screen, the subject had to hit a space bar to start recording. Due to his response latency, the subject had difficulty coordinating pressing the space bar with inspiring and beginning an utterance. The modification of a voice-activated screen sweep would eliminate this problem. In conclusion, this nonliterate subject learned to interpret the visual display provided by SpeechViewer in order to judge the accuracy of his speaking rate performance and to modify durational and loudness features of his speech behavior.

Potential To Increase Speaking Rate Although the subject demonstrated approximately a 16% increase in mean speaking rate (averaged across utterance types) from the first baseline (0.99 sps or 59 spm) to the final treatment session (1.15 sps or 69 spm), this latter rate is very slow compared to normal speakers. Because utterance tokens were randomly selected from the master pools for each session and the changing criterion in the treatment phase was the number of syllables in an utterance token, with time held constant, it was not possible to compare systematically the same utterances across treatment sessions to determine how inspiratory pause time and syllable duration contributed to changes in speaking rate. To obtain controlled and definitive measures of the relative contribution of these two factors to observed changes in speaking rate, the changing criterion across the treatment phase should be the time-base, with utterance tokens held constant. Using an alternative design such as this, information about changes in articulatory movement times and steady-state durations within syllables could be obtained by measuring formant transition and steady-state durations in the waveforms of recorded utterance tokens. However, SpeechViewer did not allow the time-base to be manipulated in fine enough gradations for this kind of design. The analyses performed suggested that both elimination of inspirations and shortened syllable durations contributed to the subject's rate increases. The subject had a maximal mean rate of 1.52 sps (91 spm) for the three utterance types, which was interpreted to be his physiological ceiling rate.

Based on this result, it was hypothesized that he had the capacity to increase his habitual speaking rate further. Visual feedback training seemed most effective for Type III utterances, whereas auditory modeling alone (baseline sessions) was not effective for Type III utterances, but was effective for increasing rate in Type I and Type II utterances.

General Comments Regarding the Treatment Procedures As the subject became more successful in eliminating within-utterance inspirations, other aberrant respiratory behaviors became apparent; for example, inspiring overly large volumes and then exhaling (losing) air, prior to initiating an utterance. To obtain more information about his speech-breathing behaviors, at the completion of the final treatment session the subject's chest wall movements and inferred lung volume displacements during quiet breathing and speech were observed using the Respitrace System (Ambulatory Monitoring Inc., 1986), connected to a storage oscilloscope. From this transducer/display arrangement, it was observed that he continued to speak without taking a quick inspiration just prior to speaking, indicating that he had not transferred his inspiratory training from the treatment sessions. He seemed to have lost this "automatic" prespeech inspiratory behavior as a result of the anoxic episode. When he did take a breath just prior to speaking, he inspired over twice his tidal volume and than exhaled about a third of this before initiating the utterance. He also continued speaking below resting expiratory level and, consequently, exerted a great deal of effort to generate phonation.

These observations highlight the importance of obtaining an in-depth understanding of a patient's speech production behavior before initiating treatment. Although the treatment procedures succeeded in eliminating the subject's within-utterance inspirations in utterances up to eight syllables, they did not address the underlying basis of his aberrant respiratory behaviors and, indeed, may have encouraged maladaptive behaviors; for example, inspiring volumes too large to control at the onset of utterance production. In retrospect, a treatment program specific to normalizing the timing and volumes of lung volume displacements during speech, across several consecutive breath groups, logically should precede the implementation of rate-training procedures.

A final consideration in judging the merit of the training procedure was its effect on the perceived intelligibility and naturalness of the subject's speech. A systematic analysis of these was not performed on the utterance tokens. A measure of the effects of treatment on perceived changes in intelligibility could be obtained using a word identification task on a randomized presentation of utterance tokens recorded during baseline and treatment sessions. Scaled ratings of naturalness could be obtained for these same items to provide information about perceived changes in speech naturalness. However, we hypothesize that the elimination of intrusive within-utterance inspirations would have a positive influence on ratings of speech naturalness, as would the increased control over vocal quality and loudness fluctuation that the subject demonstrated over the treatment sessions. We also hypothesize that intelligibility scores would remain reasonably stable over the treatment sessions, given that only a 16% mean increase in rate occurred. Elimination of within-utterance inspirations might have a positive influence on intelligibility, because listener processing of the utterance would not be interrupted by an unexpected, intrusive pause in the speech stream.

In conclusion, future directions for treatment for this subject should address modification of the subject's aberrant speech-breathing behaviors before continuing rate-training procedures. Given the subject's ability to interpret the time-by-amplitude display in SpeechViewer, he may benefit from immediate visual feedback about his success in meeting predetermined targets for speech breathing behaviors such as inspiratory locations, lung volume levels at which spoken breath groups are initiated and terminated, and coordination of expiration with phonation. This could be provided via Respitrace transducers and a throat microphone, displayed simultaneously on a multichannel storage oscilloscope. Moreover, the observation that the subject produced utterances with multisyllabic words at faster rates than those with monosyllabic words only suggests that he may be able to learn to use duration to mark syllable stress. He may benefit from specific practice to control syllable durations to mark relative stress in multisyllabic words; for example, "**p u** ppy"; "a **w a y**." Once he can do this reliably, monosyllabic word combinations could be trained using a similar stress pattern frame; for example, "**catch** it"; "a **dog**." The time-by-amplitude display in SpeechViewer could be used to provide immediate visual and auditory feedback about his success in altering syllable durations to match target stress patterns. Number of syllables in the multisyllabic words and corresponding monosyllabic word combinations could be increased as the subject progresses.

Based on these findings, recommendations for future treatment include a combination of cognitive–linguistic and motor training that incorporates immediate visual feedback to improve speech-breathing patterns and prosody. A longer term objective is to improve the subject's production monitoring skills via modeling, role-playing, and coaching, so that he can learn to adjust the length and content of his conversational turns appropriately for speaking context and conversational partners. Finally, an evaluation of the effects of these specific training procedures should include measures of speech intelligibility and naturalness in order to validate their relationship to his functional outcome for spoken communication.

REFERENCES

Ambulatory Monitoring Inc. (1986). *Respitrace systems.* Ardsley, NY: Author.

Asano, J., Ieshima, A., Kisa, T., & Ohatani, K. (1991). CT findings and prognoses of anoxic brain damage due to near-drowning in children. *Brain and Development, 23*, 227–233. (Original in Japanese. English translation available from M. Hodge.)

Berry, W., & Goshorn, E. (1983). Immediate visual feedback in the treatment of ataxic dysarthria: A case study. In W. Berry (Ed.), *Clinical dysarthria* (pp. 253–266). San Diego, CA: College-Hill.

Blackstone, S. (1990). The role of rate in communication. *Augmentative Communication News, 3*, 1–3.

Haselager, G., Slis, I., & Rietveld, A. (1991). An alternative method of studying the development of speech rate. *Clinical Linguistics & Phonetics, 5*, 53–64.

Hoit, J., Hixon, T., Watson, P., & Morgan, W. (1990). Speech breathing in children and adolescents. *Journal of Speech and Hearing Research, 33*, 51–69.

International Business Machines. (1989). *IBM Personal System/2 SpeechViewer: A guide to clinical and educational applications.* Boca Raton, FL: Author.

Kent, R., & Rosenbek, J. (1982). Prosodic disturbance and neurologic lesion. *Brain and Language, 15*, 259–291.

Kent, R., Weismer, G., Kent, J., & Rosenbek, J. (1989). Toward phonetic intelligibility testing in dysarthria. *Journal of Speech and Hearing Disorders, 54*, 482–500.

Milenkovic, P. (1990). *CSpeech* [Computer program]. Department of Electrical and Computer Engineering, University of Wisconsin-Madison, 1415 Johnson Drive, Madison, WI 53706.

Ottenbacher, K. (1986). *Evaluating clinical change: Strategies for occupational and physical therapists.* Baltimore, MD: Williams & Wilkins.

Ottenbacher, K., & York, J. (1984). Strategies for evaluating clinical change: Implications for practice and research. *American Journal of Occupational Therapy, 38*, 647–659.

Schmidt, R. (1988). *Motor control and motor learning: A behavioral emphasis* (2nd ed.), Champaign, IL: Human Kinetics Publishers, Inc.

Semel, E., Wiig, E., & Secord, W. (1987). *Clinical evaluation of language fundamentals—revised.* San Antonio, TX: The Psychological Corporation.

Yorkston, K., & Beukelman, D. (1981). Ataxic dysarthria: Treatment sequences based on intelligibility and prosodic considerations. *Journal of Speech and Hearing Disorders, 46*, 398–404.

Yorkston, K., Beukelman, D., & Bell, K. (1988). *Clinical management of dysarthric speakers* (pp. 326–352). Boston, MA: Little, Brown.

Index

Page numbers followed by "t" and "f" denote tables and figures, respectively.

251